What people are saying about …

The Hardest Peace

"Losing myself in the startling light of Kara's story, I have found who I am, who He is, and more of the meaning of every breath."

Ann Voskamp, *New York Times* bestselling author of *One Thousand Gifts*

"Kara writes honestly about a subject that few of us want to confront. She even manages to find humor in the midst of a horrifying situation. Most importantly, she points readers to the hope that is found in a God whose grace is sufficient for every trial, and whose love for His children is steadfast even in the face of despair."

Jim Daly, president of Focus on the Family

"Kara Tippetts's book *The Hardest Peace* is at the same time deeply convicting and encouraging. Kara is brutally honest in sharing her struggles all the way from a young girl to now as a mother of four battling recurrent cancer. Through it all, she has found the deep reality of God's grace and love. This is a book everyone ought to read."

Jerry Bridges, author of *Trusting God: Even When Life Hurts*

"No one chooses suffering, but everyone has the freedom to choose how to respond to it. Because she chooses Christ, Kara Tippetts can not only endure the pain and ugliness of her pilgrimage through the desert of cancer, but on the journey, she can also find beauty, wonder, joy, and even freedom from the cares of this world. By showing us how to die, Kara Tippetts shows us how to live."

Rod Dreher, author of *The Little Way of Ruthie Leming*

the hardest peace

the hardest peace

*expecting grace in the midst
of life's hard*

kara tippetts

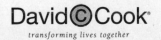

transforming lives together

THE HARDEST PEACE
Published by David C Cook
4050 Lee Vance View
Colorado Springs, CO 80918 U.S.A.

David C Cook Distribution Canada
55 Woodslee Avenue, Paris, Ontario, Canada N3L 3E5

David C Cook U.K., Kingsway Communications
Eastbourne, East Sussex BN23 6NT, England

The graphic circle C logo is a registered trademark of David C Cook.

The website addresses recommended throughout this book are offered as a
resource to you. These websites are not intended in any way to be or imply an
endorsement on the part of David C Cook, nor do we vouch for their content.

Unless otherwise noted, all Scripture quotations are taken from The Holy Bible,
English Standard Version® (ESV®), copyright © 2001 by Crossway, a publishing
ministry of Good News Publishers. Used by permission. All rights reserved.

LCCN 2014945717
ISBN 978-0-7814-1215-5
eISBN 978-1-4347-0858-8

The Team: John Blase, Carly Razo, Ingrid Beck,
Nick Lee, Susan Murdock, Karen Athen
Cover Design: Amy Konyndyk
Cover Photos: iStockphoto and Shutterstock;
family photo by Jen Lints Photography

Printed in the United States of America
First Edition 2014

4 5 6 7 8 9 10

100914

To Jason
Thank you for choosing me from all
the women in the world.

To Eleanor Grace, Harper Joy,
Lake Edward, Story Jane
Each of you has uniquely taught
me the very best of life.

Contents

Foreword

Before you begin …

Everyone has a story. While sitting in my wheelchair for more than four decades, I've heard a *lot* of heart-wrenching stories poured out in personal blogs, articles, books, or face-to-face. Sometimes, though, people who suffer become so meshed in the details they hardly see the forest through the trees—for them, trying circumstances become an inconvenient stump or a fallen log that only blocks their path to happiness. The latest medical report and PET scan are the trees of their day. They cannot see, let alone convey, the *larger* story.

It is a honed art, as well as a spiritual discipline, to be able to step back from the details and see how our own stories are woven into a much bigger one ... God's story. And Kara Tippetts in her book *The Hardest Peace* does this remarkably well.

Here is a woman who understands suffering. Her story becomes *everyone's*. You know how it is. One minute you're spiritually skipping along; the next, you're staring into the gaping jaws of affliction. Fear and claustrophobia rob you of joy, and pain becomes so disorienting you dread facing the day. Yet when night finally closes in, you pine for the morning.

When such suffering hits you broadside—as in Kara's story—you do anything to hold on to sanity. You search for someone, *anyone* who might empathize. And that's when Kara and I connected. The struggles I shared about my own battle against stage III cancer somehow reached her, and our stories resonated. She identified with me, and I with her. Perhaps that's because I've always tried to step back from my quadriplegia, pain, and cancer to understand my story in light of God's.

Kara and I both recognize that vulnerability and transparency are so *necessary* in communicating a powerful story. But we also know that our testimonies won't really reach—or even change—the life of the reader. Only the Word of God can do that. Which is why I so appreciate *The Hardest Peace*. It is filled with snippets of psalms and slices of encouraging scriptures that express the story of God and His purposes in our pain. Kara has a way of reminding us that God's reasons are perfect and that our Savior, intimately acquainted with grief and suffering, is constantly pleading our case before heaven's throne. What could be more comforting than that?

It's why I'm honored to write these opening statements for Kara's book. For we both know that suffering is a strange, dark companion; but a companion, nonetheless. It's an unwelcome visitor, but still a visitor. Affliction is a bruising of a blessing; but it *is* a blessing from the hand of God. It's why Kara calls God's peace "hard." No peace that is easy could possibly drive us into the fellowship of sharing in Christ's sufferings where we find an intimacy with Jesus that is impossibly *sweet*. So, we take suffering as though taking the left hand of God—*much* better that than not holding His hand at all.

I pray that the book you hold in your hands will inspire and refresh your heart—especially if *you* are in the midst of hardships or heartaches. Be blessed by Kara's story. For she will, indeed, help you see the forest through the trees.

Joni Eareckson Tada
Joni and Friends International Disability Center
Agoura Hills, California

Introduction

Thank you for meeting me in this place of paper, words, heart, and ideas. It is a dream to me that your eyes, or the eyes of anyone for that matter, would take the time to read something I have written. But this is even more than a dream come true; this is part of the redemption of my own story. This is my testimony of what is broken and ugly being made right and redeemed. This is the story of meeting Jesus in hard, knowing Him in today, and sharing His goodness in devastation.

I am not the first to write from the grip of cancer. I am certainly not the first to write on suffering. Many have done so before me with more clarity and understanding. I come to you in these pages as a broken woman, realizing that my brokenness may be my greatest strength—that it may be the greatest strength of us all. In the depths of my illness, I have been able to set aside my striving and look for God's presence in my suffering. My season of weakness has taught me the joy of receiving, the strength of brokenness, and the importance of looking for God in each moment.

Before cancer, I would have said I was on the journey of seeking grace, but in truth I was manufacturing my own faith. If I found a need, I did my best to meet it. My going, doing, loving was my faith, not my nearness to Jesus. In my mind I knew my efforts weren't the substance of my faith, but my practice betrayed me. Stripped of my ability, I saw Jesus in a new and profound way.

Facedown in my bed I could not manufacture anything. I couldn't serve, couldn't gather friends, neighbors, the broken to build community. I was helpless. I was a church planter's wife who could not be left alone to care for my three-year-old daughter. There were days I could not walk downstairs to join my family for a simple meal.

In those moments, I could do nothing else but begin to hunt for grace. And I found it, in the bottom of myself, my illness, my terrible. I found the Jesus who humbly washes the feet of His disciples.

Hunting for grace and living from your heart are not simple decisions. Learning the gift of each breath and spending it all in big, BIG love is the greatest calling of my remaining days—yours, too. The high calling of today is set before us both: to be humbled by the grace of God.

> But God chose what is foolish in the world to shame the wise; God chose what is weak in the world to shame the strong; God chose what is low and despised in the world, even things that are not, to bring to nothing things that are, so that no human being might boast in the presence of God. (1 Cor. 1:27–29)

This is not a book about trying to win at having the hardest story. This book is about a broken woman on the journey to know the hardest peace. Peace in the midst of *hard*. I speak both generally and specifically of hard, because hard is often the vehicle Jesus uses to meet us, point us to that peace, and teach us grace.

This is also not only a book to hand to someone who has been recently diagnosed with cancer, though I hope I could encourage many on that journey. This is a book for all of us, because all of us face the hard edges of life, whether in marriage, parenting, pain, grief, singleness … brokenness of all shapes and sizes is warmly welcomed to these pages. This is my story, but I hope it helps you look honestly at yours.

I have a few simple fears in sharing these pages. First, I fear you would hear my heart and my vulnerability and think this is how every cancer patient feels. Please resist, for that would diminish the specific journey and story of another. Each person walks uniquely in the journey of brokenness. Second, I share some of the hard edges in relationships I have faced in my life. The places where I have met discouragement and hurt have been used to cause me to move toward Jesus so He could mend my broken heart and grow in me a seeking for something bigger. So in those hard stories I present, know God is still working in my heart and in His great story of reconciliation that I may or may not see this side of heaven. It is a great hope of my heart to see it here, but I may not.

This writing has felt a bit like walking along a cliff's edge. I have put the hard edges of my story into words and felt much insecurity in the honest telling of my journey. As I write about my childhood, the messy and painful moments in ministry, the struggles in marriage and parenting, and finally the pain of my disease, I humbly entrust these words to the One who gave them. Know, dear reader, that in the hard edges of my story, I'm seeking grace and a soft heart. In the painful places of my story, I'm praying for forgiveness and reconciliation. Please do not take on an offense for me and meet any of the characters in my life's story with anything other than kindness and grace.

I realize I may not be here when these pages are bound in a book. But I trust Jesus will use them as He chooses. This is a peace I'm still struggling with.

Chapter 1

The Beginning

For everything there is a season, and a time
for every matter under heaven:
a time to be born, and a time to die;
a time to plant, and a time to pluck up what is planted …
Ecclesiastes 3:1–2

It starts as a child. I'm wrapped in fear, afraid my timid bladder will spill on the brown shag carpet. Staring at the beet-red face from little eyes, little body, little everything—the enormity of my father's anger is too big for me. He sees me struggling to hold my urine inside; he sees me weakening under his bellowing anger. This, for him, is a discipline win. He towers, he screams, he promises the fraternity paddle hanging on the wall. The brotherhood of Lambda Chi Alpha is always ready when I fall short. They are always ready to taunt me in my mistakes.

I am sent to retrieve the paddle from the wall. His paddle is always used; he's always the one to deliver the verdict, always show me my failures, always remind me of my faults. I tremble under the weight of his anger. I can feel my pee coming. I return with the paddle, and the brotherhood delivers my judgment. I crumple under the pain—it pales in comparison to his screaming. The pain came with the harsh and angry words, not the paddle. I am released first to the bathroom and then the quiet of my room to change my soiled clothes.

Anger makes us all stupid.

Johanna Spyri, *Heidi*

I am my father's daughter, raised and bruised by his anger. But that was not all. There was another in my life who taught differently, one openhearted, joyful, and brave. When I met the embrace of this woman, I felt as though I was delighted in, enjoyed, deeply loved.

Grandma Elnora. If my father was anger, she was joy. In the midst of her own, desperately hard struggles, she saw joy in simple moments like a giggle with her sisters, an ice-cold Coke held with a clean tissue, and an all-you-can-eat Chinese buffet. She loved big, instigated laughter, and was never afraid to get dirty. She extended herself in every direction to meet my siblings and me in love. She showed me how to dig worms, clean fish, and enjoy the labor of the garden. She taught me that life was seldom what you expected, but you could endure. Her hard was different from my own, but she showed me there was joy even in the harsh disappointments of life. Her farm was my sanctuary. In her home, I was the cherished granddaughter. I was the favorite, but my sister, Jonna, would tell you she was the favorite, as would my brother, Dennis. That was how big her love was, deep and wide enough to embrace us all.

The farm my grandma Elnora and grandpa Homer shared on Elliot Street was this beautiful place of peace I escaped to every summer. Endless pudding pops, cousins, watermelon served with my own saltshaker, and hours spent in search of the biggest catch in their pond. Together we would quietly wait next to one another for the subtle twitch of our bobbers. She was my hero. I wanted to grow up to be just like her, wear silky nightgowns, know where to dig the best night crawlers, and spend each extra moment in my life fishing. My best childhood memories always include her love, generous and full. I grew up wanting a kitchen painted red, scented by pork—mostly bacon—just like hers.

My home now has the stool I perched myself upon as a tow-headed young thing in the corner of my grandma's bright-red kitchen. I would sit and listen to the sweet Kentucky cadence of the accents of my family members close and distant and stories shared around her generous, full table. Plates heaped with fried potatoes, simple coleslaw, corn on the cob brought in that morning, fried fish of all sizes: bluegill, crappie, largemouth bass. Enormous sliced tomatoes partnered with loads of salt, bread and butter, and pie. I loved visiting her home; I knew the door was always open to me. I would find her running through the side door, hollering in the delight of my arrival: "Mercy, mercy, mercy, look who came to see me!" It was as though she sat waiting on her couch, peering out her picture window, looking for me.

I loved visiting there. But I did not live there.

The story of my childhood consists of high highs and low lows. Sensitive before understanding what that word meant, I struggled for footing in my littlest years. I felt my weakness; I knew my smallness. Being raised under anger, the voice of the child is lost. Seeing my brother and sister fall short grew a quiet in me that was unmistakable. The only voice I had was the one that knew how to keep harmony, be liked, and win at all costs.

I was the youngest, the observer, the witness to so much pain. I muted myself before the swelling anger that filled our house and stole the peace of all who resided within its walls. The one who struggled with anger knew the least peace. No true solitude exists when self-control is bypassed and anger given full vent. It never accomplishes its goal. When I faced my towering daddy from my smallness, his beet-red face, the spitting words at a fevered pitch, the screaming that was meant to correct only broke my heart.

It broke theirs, too. After the screaming and the paddle of the brotherhood, I was greeted by the kind faces of my siblings. They did not speak words to me, their faces a mix of relief that it wasn't them and sorrow that it was the littlest this time. We were a family unto ourselves. The only three who knew the story behind our closed doors. My brother was the oldest, my sister the middle, and then there was me. Each of us with our own unrelenting desire to please, our bond formed in pain and silence, the sibling understanding.

When my brother and sister found themselves under the heavy blow of the disappointments of our father, I would scramble to help. I remember cleaning my brother's room, mopping up the overflow of water when my sister mistakenly left the sink running. I could not make it right. I could only witness and attempt to comfort with the few tools of love I had. I could not protect them from the hard that was growing down into their own stories as their bodies grew tall.

Beyond the pain of the life we lived behind closed doors was the expectation to hide the hurt, pretend in the public moments. Let the stressed, angry one enjoy being the life of the party. We knew our roles. We knew how to look the best, act the best, use our best manners. Or we would be met with anger or silence. The truth is, my siblings and I enjoyed pleasing our parents. We excelled at it, worked at it, and lived to impress and please them. But I believe this is the story of most young children—the seeking of approval, love, and acceptance in the first place you know life.

> *I wondered who we thought we were fooling. It was as if we had*
> *all agreed upon an unspoken set of rules, a conspiracy of silence.*
> Timothy S. Lane and Paul David Tripp, *How People Change*

Eventually my siblings grew and left the house, no longer burdened under the expectation of popularity. They followed in the footsteps of my parents dutifully, joining fraternities and sororities and accepting paddles of their own, but quietly promising to never let them hang on their walls. Never be used on the little bodies they were entrusted to raise.

I walked away in stages. I believe at the age of fourteen, I stiffened my neck. My justice met its final straw, and the absence of my siblings hardened me. With my brother and sister gone from home, I no longer had the comforting connection that understood what life lived behind our closed doors was like. In their absence, a bitterness and loneliness grew in me that caused me to look for family in the connection with my friends.

I spent as much time away from home as possible. My driver's license was the greatest gift I had ever received. I became resentful to any authority in my life. I was hard, hurtful, angry, and ready to leave, but life demanded more years under the roof of the family I no longer walked in step with in private or in public. Remembering now the unkindness I lived with all those years ago hurts my heart. I hurt that my parents and I didn't have the strength of character to move toward one another. I was living with such anger, and I became an expert at pushing my parents away, farther and farther away.

I struggle telling this story, but this is the story that brought me to the end of myself. My ugly, hard heart took me down a road of desperation. I was a seeker—seeking comfort in a cheap beer, seeking to live in the laughter of the cloudy mind marijuana brought, and seeking comfort from the boyfriends who were struggling in many of the same ways as me. These young men were an attempt at running from my own reality into the comfort of the companionship of another. We were playing like adults, but as children, we didn't have the ability to navigate life with our lack of understanding. We knew precious little about life and love.

In my rebellion and anger toward my parents, I would walk in their front door and climb out my bedroom window. I worshipped at the altar of cheap beer, bad pot, and lame relationships. I was happily living on an island with my friends, enjoying utter freedom within the lies I presented to my parents. Mom and Dad were utterly connected to each other, and my problems and hardness were working at distancing them as I had hoped. I still met them occasionally at the Sandpiper restaurant to pretend and play the game that life was good—great even—if that would buy me a little more freedom.

Slowly the world I was running to became darker and darker, and my need for the escape became deeper and deeper. By my senior year, I had decided on a university solely based on the availability of drugs and parties. I chose a smoking dorm because I knew that was where the best partiers could be found. I was set to continue on this hard-hearted, dark path.

Outwardly, I knew how to play the role of life of the party; I had been trained by the best. But inwardly, I was still that little girl with urine trickling down her leg. Lost. Afraid. So very small.

By the end of my senior year, I was more than ready to leave my parents' house, the darkness within myself having become a knot. Dad and I could hardly remain in the same room together. He, taking on the new role of administrator of a school, suddenly wanted to rein me in. He was too late. I had already left. Mom and Dad found themselves hopeless at the foot of my anger, unkindness, passive-aggressive yuck. I had worn them down, worn them out, and they struggled to find places to connect with me.

But I'll never forget the day that senior year in German class, where I sat next to the zealous convert. This young Michele was beyond excited to share her story. She desperately wanted to introduce me to her Jesus. She saw my hurting heart and wanted me to meet the leaders who knew how to articulate faith. I saw in her something of Grandma Elnora: joy—joy that had nothing to do with purchased fun. Something stirred in me. Even though I had become utterly married to my bitterness, I was quietly looking for a reprieve from my spiraling story. An answer for my hurt. A truth.

I really didn't trust her, but curiosity won. Michele invited me to accompany her to youth group at Grace Community Church. That first night the youth pastor spoke on forgiveness. Not just the forgiveness available in Jesus, but the forgiveness he himself needed to live in the hard struggle of daily life—forgiveness with his wife, forgiveness to live in honest community. Ultimately he spoke of the ability to be wrong and have that wrong translated to strength rather than weakness. The public sharing of failure was revolutionary to me. Didn't this guy know these secrets were supposed to be locked behind closed doors? I could not believe he shared that he struggled with kindness in his marriage, and that he needed forgiveness to live life in love and faith. Didn't he know the unwritten rule? *Don't tell.*

I didn't have a problem seeing myself as wrong. I was simply fighting to pretend to be right in the eyes of others. This youth pastor was offering me the freedom to let all of that go. He was showing me that his weakness was his strength, and there was love to be known in brokenness. He was inviting me to open wide my hands and admit my fault, make things right, love honestly, and be loved in return. Loved, not for how I performed, but for who I was, exactly where

I was. And where I was in that season in my life was ugly, hurting, and broken.

It was more than intoxicating, this thought of living forgiven. A young woman named Jenny Gates approached me and plainly asked what I believed. She was bold and honest. She shared the gospel with me, and the message was something my heart longed for, looked for, desired. She shared how I had fallen short, but that Jesus had lived a perfect life and died the death I deserved to make me right with God, and that He rose from the dead to prove Himself God—the earth-shattering, heartbreaking, heart-mending news I was desperate for. I knew it the minute I heard it. This was different, and this was life.

Once I met Jesus, I knew my life was forever changed. But I also knew I had a lifetime of habits that I needed the grace of God to walk away from. Certainly the habits of life, but more difficult would be the anger, pride, fear, and bitterness. I knew I needed mentors and friends who would encourage me to live differently. Over time, I realized that I wanted to honor my parents and love them well, but I wanted to have the humility to live life with my future family differently. I slowly began to see grace for my parents. I desperately wanted them to know the truth of love that I was flourishing under. Unfortunately, my irritating zeal pushed them even farther away, though they were grateful to see me walking away from drugs.

At my graduation open house, I turned to my hero grandmother and asked her if it meant anything to her that I was going to be baptized. With tears in her eyes, she admitted to years of praying for me. I knew something made her love better, her food taste better, her laugh the most lighthearted laugh I had ever known. The moment I first knew Jesus, I immediately connected that this was the superpower of my beloved grandma. From this place of shared faith, Grandma and I grew closer and closer through the years. I continued to sit on the stool in the corner of her kitchen. I watched, observed, and finally understood the power of her love. It was Jesus.

My siblings and I, each in our own way, walked away from and embraced the legacy of our childhood. We all struggle to live honestly. Choosing the easier path of looking good is a constant temptation, and we all feel the inherited anger within us. The "keep quiet and look good" living is always easier than heart-baring, mistake-admitting, choosing-humility life offered in Jesus. Like our father before us, we struggle under the enormity of life and feel ill equipped to live it honestly and well. Like him, we want to rant in unbridled anger. Thankfully I have seen each of my siblings take hold of the truth of Jesus and humbly walk in repentance. The lessons were hard in coming, hard in embracing. We met much disappointment and struggle in our journey toward authentic living. For each of us, the brokenness of life exposed our need, and slowly my siblings met the prayers my grandma and I prayed for each of our family members to know Jesus. At the age of eighty-five, via my grandma's love and prayers, my grandpa came to know faith in Jesus too. Before my grandma slipped into the haze of dementia from a stroke, I shared with her the truth of faith that took hold of her husband, decades of prayers answered.

The prayer of a righteous person has great power as it is working.

James 5:16

Knowing Jesus gave me a broader imagining of life. I had been on a path of repeating what I had known, but Jesus was inviting me to live differently. I was being asked to open my heart, share my hurts, and begin to tell the story of how I lived my life behind closed doors. I was met in my hurt and loved. The secrets lived behind closed doors stopped being kept; the story of me started to develop. I blossomed knowing that Jesus was now the shining light in me, a light that gave me the freedom to be free (Gal. 5:1). The places of darkness faded. The hurt started to be released. The moments of grace and forgiveness came. I could see the knots of living that had tied up my father in anger. I could admit my own bitterness and unkindness. My heart could see and understand the quiet that enveloped my mother. My spirit could meet the two of them with love where only my own bitterness and unforgiveness had existed before.

> *To be alive is to be broken. And to be broken is to stand in*
> *need of grace. Honesty keeps us in touch with our neediness*
> *and the truth that we are saved sinners. There is a beautiful*
> *transparency to honest disciples who never wear a false face*
> *and do not pretend to be anything but who they are.*
> Brennan Manning, *The Ragamuffin Gospel*

Roles started to change, and I was granted the grace to give love in the place hurt resided. I was able to love my parents, share honestly with them, write them letters of love and forgiveness. It felt utterly miraculous. Every chance I found I told my parents I loved them.

Being recklessly loved by Jesus had untied my knots of bitterness and freed me to love in a way that was unbelievable even to me. I learned the power of our story, and began to look deeper into my parents' own story. I could not change the past, but the future could look different. Love pulsed where it previously languished. Joy began to bloom from an angry soil.

In two days, I'm returning to the *scary snort* that is a brain MRI. I call all huge tubes a scary snort. MRI, PET scans, CAT scans, radiation machines, I have met them all—every shape, every size. I remember my mom reading me the bedtime story *Are You My Mother?* by P. D. Eastman. It is a story of a little bird seeking its mama. When she came upon a huge dirt mover, she called it a *scary snort*. To me, this seems a fitting description for all these medical devices. They are big, cold, lonely, and scary, but they are necessary in this battle against cancer.

I have had so many surgeries. Under my clothes I look like a science experiment. But I am no longer the scared little girl who struggled for love. No, I enter the scary and hard looking for grace, expecting grace, with face lifted, walking in love unimaginable. Life is not as I dreamed it would be all those years ago. In many ways, it's far beyond those dreams.

My littlest daughter, Story Jane, draws pictures of me bearing multiple scars. She traces my scars with her little fingers and asks when they will leave. Story Jane rests her head on the stiff breast implants that replaced my softness and asks when I will return to my former soft self. My wounds from multiple surgeries bring her curiously close to me. Story Jane sees them, asks about them, and then lingers closely, knowing only a fraction of what they mean. I think she knows the heart of what my scars represent, but her littleness, like my own so many years ago, makes understanding our developing story difficult. I could not know the heart of my dad in his anger because of the littleness I watched from. Story also struggles to know and understand the hurt in our story from the perch of her young age. She witnesses the tears, sees my baldness. But all she knows is the warmth of my touch, here, today, and the kindness that greets her in her living. She has found new soft corners next to me that suffice where surgery has left me utterly changed. What she longs for is my closeness, my touch, my kindness to meet her each cold evening when she sneaks quietly into my bed to be near me.

She no longer asks for entrance next to me in the little hours of the night. She quietly enters by my feet and finds the warm curve in my back and returns to the comfort of her dreams next to her mama. Years will give her understanding like they gave me, but today, sitting next to my love is enough. The other day she proclaimed that she never wanted to leave my side, that I was always the warmth she liked best. I said nothing, only snuggled closer with a hope for more days. More and more days of loving her. I want her to look back and see herself a daughter of love.

Miraculously, my story had the freedom to be changed. I was able to turn over the authorship of my story to the One who knew how to best write my life. I could trust again, knowing the story wasn't promised to be easy, but I was no longer silent in it. I was a beautifully redeemed daughter of the King. I would walk in grace. But what about you? Are you avoiding your story, embracing your story, living out of the pain of your past, or looking on the horizon for Jesus to redeem your hurt and walk with you in faith?

> *He who does not long to know more of*
> *Christ, knows nothing of Him yet.*
> Charles H. Spurgeon, *Morning by Morning*

What is your story? Your real story, the story you fight to hide, the story that keeps you from freedom? The gospel frees these knots, opens truth where only silence resided. The grace of Jesus allows us to look honestly at our lives, not lock our stories into a place of shame. When I open wide my hands to the truth of my life and allow grace and forgiveness to seep into the pain of my story, I can lift my face, walk in grace and forgiveness, and not dwell on the bitter moments that hurt so desperately. It never discounts the pain. But the redemption of my hard yesterdays gives me a softened heart to walk in my tomorrows.

At the conclusion of each chapter, I will offer five questions or thoughts for you to consider. I do hope you'll take the time to think through what's being asked because although this is my story, it's also yours.

1. What are the hard parts of your childhood story?
In what ways did you try as a child to escape these difficulties?

2. Who has God sent to walk with you through your pain? Has He asked you to walk with someone else in his or her journey?

3. Consider bitterness in your heart from past hurts. Have you forgiven those who hurt you as a child? Why or why not?

4. If you could travel back in time and speak to yourself as a hurting child, what would you say? What truths did you need to hear? What truths do you need to hear now?

5. For all of us "It starts as a child." Many of the problems we wrestle with as adults can be traced back to our earliest days. Think back to my story and my hopes for my own daughter. Now think about your own childhood story and complete this sentence: I was raised the daughter or son of _____.

Chapter 2

Love Is Kind

... a time to kill, and a time to heal;
a time to break down, and a time to build up ...

Ecclesiastes 3:3

It was a cold weekend in the early part of December when I found myself with the flu, attending a weekend conference with a campus ministry of the Midwest Navigators I had just joined at college. I felt utterly awkward in their company; they consisted mostly of a very churched lot. I was desperate for a community of faith, and though we shared faith, many of them saw me as the type of person they were trying to avoid in their college experience. I showed up in my flowing broom skirt, patchouli, and thrift-shop shirt. A man there presented a ministry opportunity to those attending. In my fevered state, I heard three simple words: *mountains*, *kids*, and *Colorado*. I cornered him immediately after his talk so I could sign up and run away for the summer. I doubted I was qualified, but if desire could win someone a job, I would win.

Amazingly, I was given an interview. A gentleman called and asked me about my faith. I eagerly shared how meeting Jesus had changed my life forever and introduced me to a forgiveness I had never known—peace unmistakable. He then asked me to tell him one verse to share my faith. Just one verse. I had nothing. Silence. Crickets. I think he was stunned on the other end—*this zealous convert cannot even share John 3:16?* I gently hung up the phone, sure I would never again hear from the nice man who had interviewed me.

To my great surprise, I was offered the job as a camp counselor at the Navigators youth camp—Eagle Lake Camp—the summer of 1995. I arrived wearing a Beastie Boys T-shirt and blue Pumas. I had always loved kids, I loved the outdoors, and what state has the corner on the outdoors better than Colorado? I had no idea how "un-Christian" I looked. I had no idea how young in my faith I truly was.

That first week at staff training, everyone I saw seemed mature and deeply rooted in their faith. All the women were so gentle and soft that they looked ready to lead a sweet group of young girls going away to a Girl Scouts camp. They certainly could find the book of Amos or Galatians. They all had these packs of cards they were constantly studying. I was too embarrassed to ask what they were doing with their heads down, staring at these small cards. I soon learned the central pride and joy of the Navigators was verse memory. Memorize a verse? I had difficulty even finding a particular verse.

I was green, I looked it, I knew it, and many nights I found myself in tears. I felt like I did not belong. These people were gentle and soft-spoken; I was harsh and abrasive. They talked about their college Bible studies; I talked about the drug dealers I was sharing my faith in Jesus with. They mentioned mission trips, had CD sleeves of their favorite sermon series, and came to camp prepared spiritually to care for young campers. I came with bootleg concerts of the Grateful Dead, and the wizard sticker on the back of my car scared one of the counselors. I gave him permission to take it off, and he treated it like it would make him a leper. I felt very misplaced, but something kept me there. I knew I had a lot to learn. I secretly knew I would not end the summer looking or acting like these spiritual giants, but I sensed I was in for a sweet time of change.

My child, the troubles and temptations of your life are beginning
and may be many, but you can overcome and outlive them all if you
learn to feel the strength and tenderness of your Heavenly Father.
Louisa May Alcott, *Little Women*

I initially drove into Colorado expecting to meet a fleece-wearing, younger, vegetarian version of the Marlboro Man on every corner (minus the cigarette). Having never been west of Chicago, my imagination was the only reality in my Colorado dreaming. With the Colorado stage set, I wrote the script of my adventure. I was going west to work with kids, be surrounded by beautiful scenery, meet gorgeous men, and find my ticket out of a lifetime in the flatlands of the Midwest.

My first thought should have been a desire to be discipled and grow nearer to Jesus, but that just wasn't my heart at the time. Always the gentleman, God met me in my messy and loved me despite my poor motivations for going west. Entering the Wild West where every man was the man of my dreams, I pulled into Colorado Springs and found myself lost. I distinctly remember stopping at a 7-Eleven, expecting to see tall, brawny men drinking bad coffee, talking about their next backpacking trip. But I walked into the gas station and there were no granola Marlboro men. C'mon, where were the hunky men? I had imagined Colorado to be teaming with backpackers who loved poetry and bluegrass music on front porches, but what I found was a convenience store, a state, and a land filled with men just like the men in Indiana. Simply men working hard each day with hopes and dreams like everyone else. The Marlboro Man was created to sell something—and I had been sold. But what I found in the state was deeper, richer, better than my shallow imaginings. I had my vision of what my summer would be, but by God's grace, He had a remarkably different summer planned for me.

God was more than gracious to me that first summer at Eagle Lake Camp. He brought so many beautiful things into my life. Most importantly, he brought Shaunda. I'm not sure what she saw in me beyond a boy-crazy girl who didn't know her way around a Bible. But I guess she saw something because she became a friend who loved me in my young faith and spent hours poring over Scripture with me, showing me the beauty of my new life in Jesus. She navigated the Bible with me, showed me why everyone had their faces bent over small cards. She taught me the importance of loving the Bible and knowing it well. She helped me begin to pray. I grew hungry for things greater than my next boyfriend.

I'll never forget when Shaunda was transparent about her own weakness. Her openness with me freed me up to share my folly without judgment. In my first meeting with Shaunda, she confessed her struggles with food, how she was consumed with thoughts of a king-sized candy bar in the drawer of her husband's desk. Her vulnerability melted me. I remember turning to her after her confession and utterly vomiting all my weakness and rebellion. I told her my dating life was confusing at best, I shared my struggles with substance abuse, and confessed how I felt utterly lost in this land of spiritual giants, where it seemed no one ever struggled or failed in any way as I did. Her transparency was a freeing gift of love, and I was very hungry for more. She forever shaped how I would sit across from other young women in need of a mentor. I would always come ready to be honest, weak, and open. With Shaunda's guidance, it was a summer of amazing growth. It was also the summer I met him.

If I am going to see myself clearly, I need you to hold
the mirror of God's Word in front of me.
Paul David Tripp, *Instruments in the Redeemer's Hands*

I knew Jason that first summer only in passing. He hung with the backpackers—hiking boots, facial hair, fleece-wearing, dirty, silly, serious, and Jesus-loving. He was what I was looking for when I first arrived in Colorado. Jason would come in with two-weeks' worth of grime, play, rock climbing, and funk, and the whole package that was him took my breath away. Jason and I worked in separate areas of the camp, so I simply admired him from a distance that first summer. But then came the second summer.

I will never forget that moment, walking around the lake my second summer back in the Rockies. Praying as I hiked, I was hopeful my second summer would be a repeated time of personal growth. I had decided to return to the place that became a safe haven for me to see who I was without mind-numbing chemicals. The first summer I saw who I was without drinking and drugs, I returned to my college campus stronger in knowing myself and loving my faith. I returned the second summer expecting growth in my life beyond just stopping my fondness for living cloudy. I saw my own pride, arrogance, and selfishness. I prayed for a summer dealing with the deeper, more quiet struggles of my heart.

The second summer I still wore my Beastie Boys shirt and worn Pumas, but that summer I found comfort in my differences. I appreciated the women who had grown up in faith and didn't face the struggles I had endured. Coming back, I realized I had something to share with them. I could share the heart of the brokenhearted and challenge those women to return to their campuses and share the love they knew with someone who looked like me. I was no longer intimidated by the differences, because I knew I was uniquely made. My story mattered. I had grown in freedom and grace, and I returned not embarrassed that I wasn't a spiritual giant. I simply had more growing to do, and with the endless stream of excited campers, I had love to give.

On that first hike around the lake, praying and expecting much from my second summer, I rounded the corner to go back to the meeting hall, and I saw him. Jason Tippetts. He was walking with this strikingly beautiful woman. I remember taking a page from my friend's playbook for finding the right man, thinking, *I just need to pray her out of his life.* Maybe not the most sound theology, but I just knew there was something special about Jason. Willing to try anything, I was less than sneaky in planting myself beside him in talks and sitting at his meal table. Slowly, I wasn't having to work so hard at getting time with this kindhearted, funny guy. He started putting himself next to me. *Gulp!* Oh, and the lovely girl he was walking with ended up being his little sister. There was hope for the young convert from the flatlands of Indiana after all.

If meeting Jesus was the life changer, meeting Jason was the game changer. Jason was a young man given to gentleness, filled with a quiet strength. He enjoyed the person nearest to him, and didn't need the attention of the crowds. He connected to his campers in meaningful ways, was an excellent question asker, and had the ability to really listen—something I was desperately weak at doing. I felt heard by him, and when he was next to me, I felt like he really wanted to know my story. My real story. He was not impressed by the loud leaders who performed for praise. He was simple, honest, kind, and in all those things very complex and knowable. He was funny but could talk about pain in his life vulnerably. He communicated well and could keep up with me, a robust talker. Jason was

so handsome in his filthy, adorable, backpacker way that I was a
swoony mess around him. He once came into camp filthy from top
to bottom and asked to borrow five dollars to buy a cinnamon roll
at the bakery. I remember thinking I had never seen anyone cuter in
my life. My journal was filled with page after page of my desperate
like of this man. I could picture my life's story with him as the main
character. The thought of living beside kindness and gentleness was
not lost on me, the daughter of anger. Jason was so different from
what I had known in my childhood.

I immediately wrote home to my parents and said I had met the
type of man I wanted to marry. I was endlessly teased for this letter,
but I think my family was excited that I had made a meaningful
connection. I guess I hadn't thought a man like him existed. When
I first met Jason, I asked him what he wanted to do with his life. He
immediately said, "I'm not interested in wealth. I want to love Jesus,
and play outside with toys, loving kids and telling them about Jesus."
He set the standard for what my heart longed for in a relationship. I
didn't feel like I would ever interest him, but just knowing him had
changed me in every way. I knew my future would look different
because of him. I knew I would either be with Jason, or always be
looking for someone just like him.

But there was a hitch. I had heard from a friend that Jason
only dated within a thirty-mile radius of where he lived. I lived in
Indiana; he lived in California. I guessed I was out. So I decided to
be his friend. But he was a friend on whom I had a raging crush.
We did laundry, ate cheap Mexican food, and spent our free after-
noons reading on the beautiful lawn of a magic castle called Glen
Eryie. He read theology—Oswald Sanders, Brennan Manning,

Jerry Bridges—and I read poetry and fiction—Keats, Wadsworth, Shakespeare. We both found a literature middle ground over the book *A Severe Mercy* by Sheldon Vanauken. I was in love with the first half of the book, deeply rooted in passionate love and affection. Jason loved the second half as the couple journeyed to understand the deep theological truths of our faith. I tried to understand his deep, contemplative thoughts as he tried to understand my lofty, idealistic, poetic thoughts. We most often met in the middle: cheap Mexican food.

Much to my great delight, Jason gave up his weird, legalistic rule for dating at the end of that summer. He sat me down in a field overlooking the lake at camp and nervously asked me if I would be willing to pursue a relationship with him. I was over the moon, but instead of answering him, I pegged him with a myriad of questions: How will you honor me? What are your goals in dating me? How do you intend to protect my heart? How will we do this when it feels like there is an entire country between Indiana and California? The questions went on and on. I think I had been a bit overprogrammed in my many Bible studies. I had exactly pictured what dating would look like for us, and I needed to make sure he was on board with a dating relationship with lock-tight boundaries. I walked away and never even said *yes*. I don't know why he didn't run away right then, but he didn't. His love has always been certain. I came back to him quietly in a later meeting and simply looked at him and said, "Yes, I would love to see what is in store for us."

When we first fell in love in the dead of winter, we
said, "If we aren't more in love in lilac time,

> *we shall be finished." Be we were more in*
> *love: for love must grow or die.*
> Sheldon Vanauken, *A Severe Mercy*

We dated long-distance for a year, and then Jason moved to my college town to see how living next to each other looked. We knew camp life wasn't realistic, and long distance helped our communication—we just needed to see what daily life together would look like. After one semester together, we knew. Jason asked in December, and we said *I do* the following May. We've hit many snags and bumps, but sixteen years of marriage later, it's better than I could ever have dreamed. Jason and I married young: I was twenty-one; he was twenty-five. So we've done a lot of growing up together, the emphasis on *together*.

I distinctly remember driving away from my parents' house the day after our wedding, heading to a cabin on a lake. I was utterly silent, which is not normal for me. Jason kept sweetly asking me questions, and I would give simple, quiet answers. My mind was racing, and all that my mind kept saying was: *You are no longer Kara; you are now wife. He is no longer Jason; he is now husband. This is forever, and you had sex on your wedding night, so it's decided. He's your husband FOREVER.* I was panicked.

"Forever" felt so long and so scary. *Did we make the right choice? Did we do this too quickly like some had suggested?* Then we came to the Chicago toll road, and Jason turned to me and made one of his goofy jokes that unties all my knots. In that moment, I thought: *Thank goodness I married Jason, because he's funny, and marriage will need a lot of laughter.* I remember speaking truth into those consuming fears: *Yes, he's your husband, but look at what a great husband he's going to be. Look at the joy he brings to life. Look at him. It's going to be okay. You are so blessed to do life right next to this man.*

One of the gifts in our early days of marriage was mentors, trusted people who were safe places for us to share our ugly. For us that was Ruth and Steve, two people who loved us unconditionally and taught us the beautiful art of fighting fair in that truly hard first year of marriage. We shared the real story, not the edited, tidy version where everyone looks kind and lovely. We really shared what our lives looked like. How I often manipulated Jason to get my way, and Jason would happily let me. I would cry for flowers, then when they came, I would cry that he bought them because I cried, not because he wanted to bring them. I was a mess in the house and had zero training in keeping a tidy home. When we moved into a 675-square-foot cottage, it felt like we had 1,000 square feet of stuff. I was a terrible housekeeper. We fought over small things—it was never anything large. But those small things are huge in early marriage. Looking at them now, from where I sit today, I see how those small things were the training ground to get us through the big things.

Our mentors told us that fighting with kindness would help grow confidence in our kids. So we decided to work hard in our fighting. Our mentors talked to us about processing our last fight and talking about how we could do it more fairly the next time. Weekly they met with us and asked us about our most recent fight. They weren't looking to pick sides—they were looking for places they could encourage us to fight with more love and care the next time around. Fighting with your nearest neighbor is going to happen, but fighting with kindness? That's art. Beautiful art. Those years Jason and I spent communicating, loving, talking about the unfair way we would fight by bringing up past failures or saying the other was being like a family member, we learned the places that were unfair to speak of in fighting. Slowly, ever so slowly, the fighting became a gentle conversation between two people committed to loving each other well in the face of disagreements.

We found a safety net with our mentors Ruth and Steve. They gave us the freedom to be messy. In turn, they loved us unconditionally and helped us establish boundaries in our disagreements and fights. Our mentors taught us the beautiful art of fighting fair in that first hard year of marriage. They gave us tools to communicate well and pointed us to the redemption in the dailyness of living together.

Jason often says marriage is the fast road to sanctification. Sanctification—the beautiful and sometimes painful refining of a soul, the kindness of God to involve Himself in our growth in grace. Marriage is often the beautiful tool He uses to shape our lives and expose our edges. He uses the hard edges of our living, grows in us forgiveness and the joy of repentance, and teaches us the beauty and gravity of unconditional love and its ability to grow the object of our love in amazingly beautiful directions we never expected. Identifying expectations and idols we both lugged around about what we imagined marriage to be, facing the reality of what it actually was, and honestly looking at those painful, unmet expectations and moving toward each other in love and forgiveness was the hardest living and learning we both had to do in those young married years. Motivations to hurt were rarely there, but so often our expectations were unmet and tender and led to our most difficult fights.

This is indeed the deepest comfort—to be accepted by God, totally forgiven, and then by grace to forgive the deepest wounds and hurts.
Rose Marie Miller, *From Fear to Freedom*

My dear friend put it well when she said, "We all carry around within ourselves a cage of rats." The rats are our unkindness, our sin struggles, tensions our personalities bring, and our hardness of heart. We know these rats well. We love some of them, and we hate some of them, but ultimately we work very hard at hiding them from those who know us. We are quietly testing the boundaries of the depth of love in our relationships. For me, it felt like marriage became this moment when I could release the rats—those early years were a testing of Jason's unconditional love. Not only did he get my morning-grouch rat, he got my slob-in-living rat, my panic-hateful-clean-up-this-mess-someone-is-coming-over rat, my please-always-say-exactly-what-I-want-you-to-say control rat. Oh, my blessed, gentle husband looked all my ugly rats in the face and said, "Kara, I love you—rats and all. You are mine for always." And slowly, I trusted him. I believed his love, and we worked on the rats. God loves us the same way, but He loves us in such a way that says, "I have something better. I can change your heart. I'm not afraid of your rats, but I have a greater joy than these silly, hateful creatures that steal the best of life from you."

Do I still have rats? Certainly. Do I use them to fight unfairly? Sometimes, yes. But I know something much greater. I know living next to my guy in gentleness and love is one of the greatest gifts I have known this side of heaven, and I want to live and treasure that love. I want to move past my own unkindness with love, and know the reckless love of Jesus, and extend that love—that unconditional, always-believing-the-best, full-of-forgiveness-and-grace love. There are days when love abounds, and days I cannot find it. But when I'm looking upon my love, the lover of my soul, my eyes grow more clear in my calling to love my guy with all the love I have to give.

Disclose rather than be exposed. We will be exposed anyway when we see Jesus face-to-face. We might as well do it now.

Ed Welch, "Disclose or Be Exposed," Christianity.com

None of us realizes how before marriage we spend our little years, our teen years, and especially our college years dreaming, envisioning, creating ideas of exactly what marriage will be and the multiple ways it will heal our hurts, brokenness, and loneliness. We begin to look closely at marriages and relationships we desire to emulate, and we begin to prescribe for ourselves the perfect marriage. In essence, we create a golden calf idol of the many ways marriage will *fix* us. But marriage was never designed to fix.

It didn't take long to realize the enormous idol Jason and I had created in these longings and dreams. No matter how kind and loving the person you marry is, there will always be a void. I often tell my friends looking at my marriage from the outside that, as good as he is, Jason could never cure my loneliness. There are moments and glimpses, but truly the most intimate place in my heart is reserved for Jesus. No matter how hard I try to fit Jason into that space—and trust me, I've tried—he simply won't fit.

Marriage, for me, was the place I first really saw my selfish heart. Living in friendship I could take my grouchy moments and hide them away alone in my bedroom. Marriage never seemed to afford me very much privacy from my own unkind struggles. Marriage is a beautiful unveiling of the real me—no hiding. That is scary, and that is amazing.

I distinctly remember the impact of a particular man I heard speak years ago. At the time, I was working as a fourth-grade teacher at a private Christian school, and one of the local pastors came and spoke to the kids. He shared his childhood story of having a painful stutter, a mouth full of braces, and being very small compared to other children in his class. This grown man spoke vulnerably and tenderly about the pain he had endured as a young boy. His pain ran deep, and it had shaped who he became. The honesty with which this man spoke touched me deeply. He asked the children to focus on three simple words: *Love is kind* (1 Cor. 13:4). There are times when things change us in a very sudden way. Hearing those three simple words suddenly changed the direction and focus of my life. I was pregnant with my first baby and still wading through the struggles of our new marriage. It dawned on me: Could these three simple words make a difference in all of life? Could these words, used by the Holy Spirit, effect real change in my life and the relationships around me?

This gentleman's message was a profound addition to the hard work Jason and I had been doing with our mentors. They had challenged us that explosive fighting would create insecurity in our yet-to-be-born children, and this greatly motivated us to do the hard work of learning to fight fair and communicate honestly. In other words, to be kind.

Love is kind. Those three words became the foundation for our marriage. There may be no greater truth or challenge. But we were about to experience how those three words came into play with the birth of our children.

The spring after I heard that life-changing message, our first baby girl was born. I looked into her beautiful face and knew immediately I was going to name her for my dear grandma. Eleanor full of Grace is the name I gave my first daughter. Eleanor for the woman who showed me unconditional, big love, and Grace for the church where I first heard of Jesus. She was followed by three siblings: Harper my Joy, Lake Edward, and Story Jane. All named from rich places of meaning and seasons of grace. With each child, the effort at living in kindness grew more important and more difficult. My heart longed to live behind closed doors without hiding, without shame, without bitter anger when the edges of each ordinary day are deeply felt. The little years of babies, young children, life, and work can stretch one unbelievably thin; the hard edges of each moment were felt, the anger close to the surface. Money is tight, sleep is short, needs are great, and there never feels like enough Mama or Daddy to fulfill the needs of growing children.

The challenge of living in kindness was and is a lofty calling. Jason and I partnered in every way in those little years. They were exhausting years, but we were committed, even at our most exhausted, to parent with kindness. We helped each other, loved each other, and gave each other time when exhaustion met its max. And when we failed, there was repentance—the quiet turning to the person we hurt and asking for forgiveness and praying for Jesus to help us to change. Simply change our hearts, but there is nothing simple about it.

Sleepless nights, seminary, an utter heartbreak with church, we clung to Jesus and worked daily on loving each other well and with kindness. We went through a very difficult season when Jason finished seminary. We faced hard hearts, sin, and unkindness within the church, and God used it to grow us in our love and boundaries in our life. God used that hard to show us the fruit of the years of working on our relationship.

The heartbreak of church? Well, it was a place I had imagined we would spend the rest of our days ministering to and loving a small community, a place in the Blue Ridge Mountains. God had a different plan, though, and it took heartbreak to move us on from our own ideas. We are often too stubborn and willful to be moved any other way. We hold tight to what we think the plan is, and God must be sovereign in His planning. Our tight grip made this hard, particularly for me. I put my roots down deep and felt the pull of the place to remain forever. I dreamed of life shared with a people, and one day—maybe one day—my dream of a farm just like my grandparents'.

We gave our lives for nearly eight years to a small mountain town. In those precious years, the years babies are born and life is lived in the chaos of little ones, I fell utterly in love. God grew a contentment in me in a place where the pace is slow, the accents unique, and the food rich and mostly fried. I remember sitting with a man who had grown as dear to me as my grandpa. I sat at Jack's feet, and we both knew his days were numbered. Together we held hands and wept. We shared how thankful we were for each other. Fears at sharing love vanished as he knew he was about to depart. He was brave in blessing me in my days to come. We shared the moments of joy that we had been able to live beside each other. His heart was ready to go home, and we talked about that journey. He flew away to Jesus before he saw what happened to the church he spent a lifetime loving. The call came that he breathed his last, and I immediately traveled to sit beside his love of over sixty years. I held her hand and spoke no words. There was present grace in that moment, and there was deep sadness. When you walk through these dark valleys with another, a family, a community, you cannot see beyond those shared moments and imagine a living beyond them. I sure didn't want to.

Soon after Jack flew away, there was a defining moment when we knew we were not meant to stay. We saw a lack of willingness to do the hard work of facing pain and admitting fault in the firing of a man who had served the community for years. One person decided he was utterly opposed to us remaining. We were not surprised by the unkindness of this one, as he had done terrible damage in previous churches. What did surprise us, though, was the lack of courage in confronting him in favor of the easier road of moving on and forgetting. We were deeply grieved, but felt we were given the grace to walk away from an unhealthy situation.

Jason wanted to protect the hearts of our children from the pain of such unkindness, so we made the brave and impossible decision to leave. It was made harder in leaving without knowing what was coming next. We returned to a small home we owned on the other side of town. We put a tire swing in the backyard, and we started to enjoy watching the sun set. We taught a child to ride a bike; we enjoyed fires and cooking together. We learned a new exhale we had not felt in a long time. There was no one to please, no winning, no expectations, just us. It was a quiet time, a sad time without too many words, and it was a healing time. The children had our focus, and we had time to reflect and see God's goodness in the midst of pain in a new way.

I named my youngest daughter for that community of faith. When people ask where her name—Story Jane—came from, I tell a story of love. I speak of a place where much of my heart still resides. I do not regret naming her for a place that caused so much pain. I see how much of the pain was my own tight grip, my inability to trust Jesus, my longing for love. No, as I pray for the place that I proudly named my daughter after, I believe God is bigger. He was for me, and I pray He will be for them.

In the impossibility of walking through this season of life, I remember clinging to Jason at night and asking him if we were going to be all right. It felt like our hearts were going to break and never again heal. He turned to me and gently told me, "Kara, tomorrow we get to wake up and be faithful. Whatever each step brings, and whatever hard comes, people will always disappoint us. But tomorrow, tomorrow we get to be faithful in that moment." I remember trusting him, loving him, and knowing we would truly be kept that day and the days that would follow. Sometimes the hardest peace to find is the peace in saying good-bye and leaving the work of justice and reconciliation to Jesus. It was a peace slow in coming, but it came. We were given the grace to leave, to drive away, to move to the land where the mountains are tall, the food different in every way, and the community utterly different but equally beautiful.

The work of restoration cannot begin until a problem is fully faced.

Dan Allender

When I look at the multiplying gray hairs in the beard of my love, the years feel like they have so quickly overtaken us. Beside the lake at camp, we were baby-faced idealists with a horizon of tomorrows to enjoy. Those three words—*Love is kind*—have drawn us together in a way that allows us to face each new hard. We never knew what the education of kindness would be called on to walk through in our days beyond the pain faced in ministry. Jason never expected to learn the art of loving a shell of my former self in the devastation of disease, and loving without love being returned by his cancer-quieted wife. The education of kindness came when, night after night, Jason found me in bed, drugged, weepy, and unable to help in the home in any meaningful way. Jason learned the value of kindness as daily love was delivered to our door through meals, cards, endless kindnesses. It was the grace that carried us, nourished us, and reminded us of goodness.

We learned the high calling of kindness when the horizon of our days was taken from us, giving us uncertainty. We have walked in kindness when it felt like the only thing we could manage. God led us with gentle love and we followed, quietly, broken—we followed. We subtly move in our days toward each other. The moving is easier some days, but the effort of moving toward each other is never lost. Our love story has grown deep in our pain, in the pain we never expected. We never realized the deepening in our story would carry us through an endless rotation of appointments that leave us utterly broken and clinging to each other.

Jason and I met young-faced and wanting to be the best at marriage. We wanted to win. We worked, we struggled, we fought for honesty in our community to learn to love each other better. I have this enviable marriage now only because we walked through and not around the hard in our marriage. We learned to look past annoyances and look at loving the heart of the other. I still grow annoyed when Jason wads the wet washcloth in the corner of the bathtub instead of spreading it out over the faucet or the side of the tub, but those small irritations don't keep me from moving toward Jason in love and kindness.

This past year has taught us that winning at marriage isn't what we thought it was. We thought it was being safe together, loving each other in kindness, and meeting the other in moments of ugly with grace and forgiveness extended. We thought it was gentleness and affection. We were admired for our love spent over coffee and in prayer. Our marriage, full of support and tenderness, was a landing place for many hurting marriages. In a way, we were winning at marriage. But I remember the moment Jason came home this year from an Acts 29 conference. He was quieted by a truth that had impacted him deeply. Before he left for this trip, tumors were found in my uterus, and we were expecting cancer's return. He said someone was sharing how really loving God meant withholding nothing. I was in our bed looking at him, and he looked at me and wept. I didn't need to ask him. I knew the deep question of his faith that was being asked. Would he open his hand and withhold nothing, even me?

He is sleeping deeply beside me now. The ebb and flow of his breathing is a comfort. I have been battling a fever for a week. There was a fever before this one and some pain. I want to wake him with my tears to have him comfort me and tell me it's not cancer's return, but I know he's weary from the day of doing both of our roles—Mama and Daddy. And at the heart of marriage, he can love me, he can hold me, he can comfort and walk next to me through the valley of the shadow of death, but he cannot save me. So tonight, maybe this once, I will let him sleep. My Savior is not unaware of my pain and fear of cancer's return.

Consider your love story. Or maybe the lack of one. How do you expect a human love story to save you where it cannot? What are the unfair expectations you place on that relationship? Do you use the rats within yourself to hurt the ones you love most? Do you see another marriage you admire? If so, think about sharing a meal with that couple. If they are transparent and open about the struggles and victories in their life without speaking unkindly about each other, consider asking them to mentor you in your marriage.

1. How has kindness shaped your life? How has the absence of kindness left you broken?

2. Where do you see grace working on your heart to help you love an unlovely person like Jesus loves the unloveliness in you? Kindness is a gift given and received when we don't deserve it. Romans 2:4 says, *God's kindness is meant to lead you to repentance.*

3. Can you recall a time when you did not fit in but someone reached out in kindness to love and accept you? What impact did that kindness have on you?

4. If you are married, what are some expectations you had going into marriage that were not met? How did you reconcile those unmet expectations? How has God shown you that only He can satisfy you fully?

5. Do you fight with kindness? What would that look like? How would your relationships change if your fights were rooted in kindness?

Chapter 3

The Unexpected Plot Change

"A time to …"

In the early years of our marriage, a small book swept the Christian community. It was *The Prayer of Jabez* by Bruce Wilkinson. It was one of the fastest-selling books of all time. It was a simple book that found a small verse tucked within the confines of a giant narrative found in 1 Chronicles 4:10: Jabez called upon the God of Israel, saying, "Oh that you would bless me and enlarge my border, and that your hand might be with me, and that you would keep me from harm so that it might not bring me pain!" One could walk into most any church and find banners emblazoned with this verse. People begged this prayer, proclaimed this prayer, and the book was a sensation. We all wanted giant borders without pain. It was a season of plenty. We had a copy of this book, and I am certain this prayer passed through our home, from our own lips. We liked what this prayer seemed to offer—plenty without pain. Who didn't want the offerings of great borders and no suffering?

Then all at once, everything changed. That September day happened, four airplanes meant for harm destroyed buildings and lives and so much more. And overnight the book vanished. The banners of great wealth and endless borders were taken down. Gradually cynicism took root, and the luster of more started to fade. But quietly, ever so quietly, I'm not sure any of us let go of that small prayer.

As Jason and I walked through our story, we noticed we weren't winning by the world's standards or even the church's standards. But in the "losing," we were finding a richness we could not quantify. We were finding ourselves restored in the midst of our brokenness.

Recently, as I remembered this small book that swept the nation, I asked Jason a simple question: "What if our story had happened in the time of this book and the gluttonous prosperity of that season?

Would we have had a place for our story to reside, or would the winning of that day have shamed us?"

I grieve my own thirst for comfort, ease, plenty without pain. I wonder whose story I didn't hear back then in that Jabez season. I would be lying if I said I still don't long for those extended borders in my life and the absence of pain. But what if that prayer was meant for Jabez and simply for Jabez? Maybe the part of the prayer that is meant for each of us is that God's hand might be *with us*. And simply that. I am not accusing the prayer of Jabez as being a false, unfair prayer to pray, but I think we should all be honest with our love of that verse. We all wanted more and ease, and we wanted to use God to get it.

But we are not the Author of our story. We are the characters.

By the mercies of God, an opportunity opened up for us to plant a new church in a place we held dear—Colorado. The heartbreak of our former church taught us ministry is never neat and tidy. It can be good, and some days very good, but it is rarely clean. With that lesson fresh in our minds, we hoped to plant a church not of prosperity but of honesty. We simply had no idea how honest it would be.

We decided to beat the movers by one evening. We were eager for our new town, and a beautiful friend had organized a campout in our short-term rental: a fire and sleeping bags and simple food. We were road weary, but so thankful to finally be home. The kids explored the place, and then we settled down for bed about eight thirty that night. I remember falling asleep so quickly. Around ten I woke up, and not wanting to wake the kids, I ran up the stairs to use the bathroom. Dehydration, altitude, exhaustion—it all hit me like a ton of bricks. I remember thinking, *I'm going to throw up*. I stood from the toilet to turn to vomit, and that's the last thing I remember. I woke a short time later with my face in a pool of blood and in desperate pain. Jason was there calming me, assuring me.

My teeth had gone through my lip, and I had broken my nose in two places. My face was the only thing to break my fall on the cold, rough tile. Jason got me to the hospital, and because I had passed out, the doctor said I must have a CAT scan and EKG. So I was admitted. This was not how I imagined our first evening in our brand-new, hopeful town.

I looked at Jason anxiously after we learned my heart was not in rhythm and said he could not stay in the hospital with me, that we simply could not let our kids wake up in a new town to strangers and their mama in the hospital. Besides, the movers were coming in less than five hours. Alone in that hospital room, in a brand-new town, I remembered a question I had asked a group of young girls I had worked with: "In the absence of comforts and friends, is Jesus enough?" In that cold, stark hospital room, with only employed staff as my company, that question echoed through my mind. The answer was sure and the peace was present. It was an answer I was holding tight.

What followed were months of tests and needing/getting a cardiologist at the age of thirty-six. We waded the waters of heart monitors and figured out why my heart went awry that cold night in January. My nose healed, as did the bruises, and the stitches were removed from my lip. It was determined that the fall is what sent my heart into A-fib. We rested in that good prognosis and dug into church planting. We were meeting people, hosting dinners, speaking in community groups, and sharing our vision for a simple, honest, gospel-centered church on the west side of Colorado Springs.

Still, my fall humbled us and changed our perspective. What if it wasn't a mistake that I was brought to town to start our journey in ministry as a *broken* woman? What if our journey was intimately planned to be hard, and that story is the good story? What if the glow of prosperity isn't a glow at all but a unique stink? What if suffering isn't to be avoided but received and embraced?

We determined our desired location for a home and began our house hunt. One day, after dropping the kids at school, we happened upon an estate sale. I kept looking past the items for sale and noticing the house. There was a huge cottonwood tree in the backyard that reminded me of North Carolina—it was made for a tire swing. I turned to Jason and said, "This is it." And it was, a perfect house with more guest rooms than we needed. We did not understand why we would need two guest rooms, but then again, we did not know the path that would unfold for our family.

On a Saturday evening, after our first week in this perfect, new house, a fire started in what is known as Waldo Canyon. It is a place I had often passed but never visited. This canyon is near to our perfect, new house, the house we could not wait to move into, where we would meet our neighbors and begin to dream the honest church that would start to form on the west side of town. That fire started on Saturday, and by Tuesday evening our house found itself in an evacuation zone.

We mostly lived in disbelief that this fire would actually have anything to do with us. Most evenings we would sit together, read updates from news sources, and watch the smoke on the ridge. We had fascinating views of wildlife, but we felt completely separate from this fire. Sure we packed, we videoed our belongings, we prayed, but we just didn't believe we would be displaced, evacuated, sent away.

That Tuesday we decided to take the kids to a movie in an actual movie theater. We forked over the money to see *Brave*, but what we were really there for was to get a break from the heat and the constant coverage of the fire. We had our dear friend Erika visiting, and we LOVE a good movie. While we were inside enjoying the movie, the winds outside shifted, and everything about that fire up to that point changed. As I came out of the theater, I looked to the sky and saw the largest smoke plume I had ever seen. As I rounded the corner of the mall, the entire ridge was in flames. My heart sank. I tried to keep composed for the kids, but I could hardly function. As I drove toward our new home, all I could think was, *I'm going in the wrong direction. Why am I driving toward this mess, this chaos, this horror? I need to be going in the opposite direction.* I had phoned Jason and he was equally stunned. We met at home and had maybe fifteen minutes to pack, give our possessions that are dear to us to friends, and leave before the smoke was so oppressive that we couldn't breathe. Erika worked hard to keep the kids calm as I frantically packed the most random assortment of clothing I have ever packed. I packed myself maybe one and a half outfits. Our stress was as thick as the oppressive smoke. We knew we had to go, and go quickly. I grabbed pictures, journals, childhood memories, and love letters. It was all that had value to us when we were only given minutes to decide what was most important.

Ten days before, we had rented a twenty-six-foot U-Haul to carry our belongings to our new home. Ten days later, we found ourselves driving down the road with our children, Erika, and a very few belongings. Those endless things that filled our giant moving truck suddenly lost their value. They became things, whereas the people next to me became my treasures. The contents of the relationships in our car were the things that mattered. As we drove away, the children were happily playing in the backseat. They were together and they barely noticed the nightmare on the ridge. But Jason and I felt the burden of driving down the road without a destination, fleeing a scene I still cannot describe in words but will never, ever forget. Had the movie *Brave* lasted thirty minutes longer, we would not have been permitted home to pack the few belongings we took—the scattering of clothes, our love in letters, pictures, and a few items that feel important and sentimental when you have merely minutes to decide.

We drove into Colorado with visions in our heads of how hopeful things would be. The reality that greeted us was a broken nose, blood, heartache, and the west side of our new town literally on fire—the side we had chosen as our own.

Do you not see how necessary a world of pains and troubles is
to school an intelligence and make it a soul?

John Keats

That fire pried our hands from our things. It took the moments of intense smoke, devastation, and fear to show us the contents of our car were the only contents that mattered. In other words, people. Many people lost their homes in the Waldo Canyon fire, one of the worst in recorded Colorado history. We did not, and after a time we were allowed to return. We reentered our home that I had spent hours of my life on Pinterest imagining beautiful and put-together, and realized the orderly, decorated, crafty corners no longer held the luster they had just one week before the fire. The fire showed me the meaninglessness of our stuff in a new way. Certain perspectives had been burned away. Don't get me wrong—if it had all burned, there would have been intense grief and sadness for everything I had forgotten to grab, but the relationships that remained and the relationships that grew as a result of that fire are what matters.

Two weeks later, the kids were playing, I was cleaning smoke damage, and it came time for me to get ready for the date Jason and I had planned. In the midst of a shower, I decided I needed to do a self–breast exam. I just sensed that I needed to. As soon as I started, I knew. I found the hard mass and started to cry. I called Jason, crying. I called a friend, crying. I just knew.

We sought out the proper doctors, the surgeons, the oncologist, and our fears were confirmed on a blazing hot summer day. July 23. A day that forever shaped our family. The radiologist told us he was almost certain I had cancer. He told us to see a breast surgeon as I needed to have significant surgery. The moments I remember about July 23 are only bits and pieces. We did not expect the pathology of my biopsy to have come in so quickly. The breast surgeon sat down and looked me straight in the eye: "I have seen the report from your biopsy, and you do, in fact, have cancer." From that point, I felt like Charlie Brown in school. *Wahh, wahh, wahh … mastectomy … wah, wah, wah … You will lose all your hair … wah, wah, wah … aggressive cancer.* I kept looking at my dear friend Anna, who we had brought along to take notes. With tears in her eyes, she was frantically writing. She kept telling me she was getting it all. She was a nurse and familiar with the terms, the words, the plan, but she had to look through her own tears and shock to place the pen to the paper.

From the point the doctor confirmed cancer, I could not take in any other words coming out of her mouth. They were septic, clinical, and I simply looked at her short auburn hair while tears streamed down my face. She spoke with confidence about my next steps, but I was more crumpled than the paper I was sitting on in her stark office. She came to my side to show me the devastation cancer had already had on my breast. The visual on her iPad was so hard to stomach. She grabbed my nipple, pointed out how it was dimpled, and said, "This will have to go." She had seen hundreds like my own, but I was looking at my breast utterly new. It had nourished the lives of my little ones, and now it was looking at me like a guilty stranger trying to kill me. In her hand, she was the mechanic telling me my fuses were bad, but they weren't fuses. They the life-giving part of my being—they were utterly connected to me.

We left the office and sat in the car for a very long time and cried. All three of us just wept. I said I wanted to meet with our pastor, Mark, but he was at lunch. So we all decided to go to Whole Foods and buy something to eat. Isn't that what you do when you have cancer, decide it's time for Whole Foods? I wandered the aisles and found some berries and water. They were tasteless, sour at best, my own grief making their amazing summer freshness taste sour and awful. The tears continued as we met later with our pastor and his wife. We prayed and simply shared what information we could piece together from our meeting. My sweet note taker, Anna, called our medically minded family members who wanted specifics. I remember calling my father-in-law, Ed, who is so dear to me. He could not even speak. He actually hung up on me in his grief.

This was not the story I had planned.

The fire stole my thirst for stuff, the things of life. And cancer stole my moments, replacing them with an intensity to live every breath with intention. I loved before cancer, I shopped before the fire, but both of these devastations brought with them a new filter through which we saw all of life. We often called it our new normal that didn't feel at all normal. We stumbled in those first days to know how to live, to remember to eat, and to find life in the midst of our horror and diagnosis and stress. I would bathe my little ones and feel the impossibility of what we were about to face with such young children. But, as Jason said in the Blue Ridge Mountains, each day we were given we had the privilege to fight to be faithful in it. We simply didn't know what that faithfulness would look like, but we trusted Jesus to be gentle in teaching us the footing.

We thought we would come to town, present our strength, love big, and begin to build a small tribe of believers who would share Jesus with this community. Instead, we came to town broken by a fall, set on edge by a fire, and stripped of strength with cancer. We felt like the little drummer boy, only able to offer a drum filled with weakness and need. That's all we had, that and Jesus. Our new church community was shaped from the very beginning by our brokenness. To their credit, they welcomed us, loved us, and became a safe place where we could be at the end of ourselves. When you come to the end of yourself, that's when something else can begin. And what began for us is that we started asking for help. We had to. People say as the leader goes, so goes the organization. I believe the same can be said about a church. Our church became a place to show up needy. We had to let go of our false comforts found in control and strength. We said yes to offers of care and help. We stopped pretending we had anything figured out. Cancer stripped us of that pride. We simply asked for our daily bread, to get through each moment, for Jesus to carry us and meet us in our daily mess. We began to experience the church we had always dreamed of. We just never expected it to come through our own brokenness.

Our family all around the country partnered in providing the funds to hire a housekeeper. Our community stocked our refrigerator and brought us nourishing meals and lunches for the kids to take to school. A friend even came each week to bring fresh flowers, and her daughter cleaned out my refrigerator of the many different containers that had found themselves moldy and stinking. I remember watching this young girl opening lids and sniffing suspicious containers and feeling specifically loved because smells were especially hard for me after treatment. Someone even noticed a clunky appliance and had a new one delivered. Our needs were met before they could even be spoken.

Friends came and quietly sat beside my bed and allowed Jason to take the kids out to dinner on my darkest days. My littles witnessed so much of my frailty that they needed time away. Having my feet rubbed distracted me from my nausea that was intense. So a parade of humble servants came to my bedside and loved me as they rubbed my feet and listened to my struggles while the family ran away to laugh and forget, if only for a moment. They needed the safety of one another and favorite things like Mexican food. Friends from all over the country flew in, bringing love to our home. *Humbling* is the only word. Jason and I decided early that we needed people to move in with us to help manage our home with four young children. Several women came, my brother and sister came, and my dear friend Mickey even gave us three months of her life so my family could be cared for. Mickey created a haven of safety in our home that surrounded my children in one of the darkest seasons of my treatment. One evening Jason turned to me and said now he understood why God made sure we had two guest rooms in our new home.

When we lay the soil of our hard lives open to the rain of grace and let joy penetrate our cracked and dry places, let joy soak into our broken skin and deep crevices, life grows. How can this not be the best thing for this world? For us? The clouds open when we mouth thanks.

Ann Voskamp, *One Thousand Gifts*

I could not wait for my health to return to fully participate once more in life. I longed for simple moments cooking and dancing with my children. I longed to do the school driving and attend sporting events. I wanted to hike, bike, to live apart from the facedown living I had been doing in my bed for months. We were so ready. Summer came, and we went on a long vacation. We played hard; we rested hard. We reconnected after weeks and weeks of feeling unraveled. It was a glorious summer. I would wear out quickly, but I was so happy just to be alive.

I had one more procedure I needed to complete, then I was going to make strides at battling cancer with my diet and a naturopathic doctor as well as my team of regular doctors. The last step in my aggressive approach was to have my ovaries removed. My type of cancer encouraged this. I went for a consult with a specialist in the field, and he agreed about the removal, but he was hesitant to take my uterus. He did not want to overtreat me, so he decided to do an exam. What he found were more tumors. And I found myself facing more tests.

I was forced into a radical hysterectomy. I woke from the lengthy surgery to hear my prognosis was the worst possible outcome: breast cancer had returned, or maybe it had never really left. My heart was weary. I did not feel up for another battle with cancer. Jesus knew the prayer of my heart was something like a Jabez prayer, that I would not have any more cancer, that the pain would go away. But that's not what He's promised. It is His presence that is sure, so I trust Him. I have trusted Him. I will trust Him. When I told my firstborn what might be, she simply said, "Mom, we know how to do this." She was right. We have a Good Shepherd; we do not travel this road alone.

The diagnosis came and my case was passed around by multiple doctors. They were honest about how my story grieved them. They hated seeing the young women coming through their office with such painful stories. From the moment I looked at my mammogram, I knew it would be hard for me to ever escape my battle with cancer. The picture of my cancer was all tentacled, my breast a snow globe of calcification. In those first moments of "seeing" my cancer, I knew the battle I was about to face would be fierce—one that I might not win.

I admitted having headaches. I won an MRI, and it indicated cancer had entered my brain. I called Jason with the news. He drove home to find me crumpled in the corner of my room, hopeless, afraid, uncertain. I'm not sure if you know this, but the words *brain* and *cancer* used in the same sentence are no joke. It seemed ridiculous. Impossible. Hopeless. We immediately met with doctors of every brand: radiologist, neurologist, oncologist. They offered confident solutions, and they whisked me into treatment that very hour. I was introduced to a scary snort I aptly named *the stink eye*, and was shot with eighty-nine targeted blasts of radiation that met my tumor within a tenth of an inch. Hope felt somewhat restored, though the reality of cancer entering my brain left a wound that caused us to struggle to trust.

We initially thought the treatment was harmless. But soon I was losing words, forgetting, and struggling to accomplish tasks. I started arguing with Jason over conversations he said we had. I quietly knew he was telling the truth, but I didn't want to admit to another weakness. After another tense conversation of forgetting, I finally broke. I admitted the change in my sharpness and ability to recall and remember. Jason gently agreed and grieved, telling me the change he had witnessed in my mind. I finally spoke to my doctor with honesty about my struggles. He said it was a combination of treatment and the hormone suppressants that were sending me into ultra old-lady menopause, that for young women this drug was staggeringly difficult.

All this to say, life is nothing like the one I imagined as a little girl sitting in my grandma's kitchen. My story has had a plot change I never expected. Actually, it's been more of a plot *twist*, that word being much more descriptive of how it's felt. No one ever imagines disease, heartbreak, and horror in their story. We always imagine health, wealth, winning, blissful joy—the stuff on which the Jabez prayer is built.

Being public about my cancer, I often have people admonish me for calling it *my* cancer or speaking so frankly about my battle with cancer. As if speaking the language of my disease is somehow making it an ongoing reality. How limited would God be if my honesty about my disease was His limitation to cure it? That would be an impotent God I would really like little to do with. But the God I know, the sovereign God of the Bible, knows well my story of suffering and offers Himself at every turn. If the honesty with which I tell my story were the limitation of His strength, well, I would be utterly screwed. But imagine if He were intimately involved in my story, which He is. Imagine if he showed Himself in my hard, which He did, and what if the hard of my story is the beautiful redemption of my today? Could suffering then take on a different hue? Could the coloring of the hard not be so dark, so hateful and gloomy? The well-meaning emails that admonish the way I speak about my story cause me to wonder at the depth of grace that can be understood without the presence of God in the midst of our suffering. If our hard is the absence of a good God, then how can anyone walk in faith?

I spent the holiday season this year after my second and third diagnoses looking deeply into the faces of the ones I love most. I longed to remember what it was like not to count my days, to be lost in the bliss of ignorance of how much remains. With every action I wondered, *Is this my last Thanksgiving, my last meal of mostly brown shared with people I love, like, and desire close? Are they counting my Thanksgivings? Did they feel bound to accept my invitation because of cancer?* I know cancer is what brought people pilgrimaging from states and states away. I'm a decent cook, but it was cancer that brought everyone close—not my gift for sugar-free baking.

Counting. Yes, my cancer forces me to count. And so I do. Days, holidays, moments, breaths—all of it this strangely beautiful gift of noticing each moment. I can tell when I look in Jason's eyes that he's counting too. I see the hunger in him for more breaths, more time for our feet to touch in the night. He wants to prolong the conversation he dreads. He loses his breath thinking of the moment he has to tell the kids I'm not there for the wiping of tears, signing of permission slips, telling of stories, toasting of bagels, picking of dance party songs—that he has to shoulder it all. He knows he can; he simply doesn't want to do it—he isn't that fond of dancing.

I see the dread in his eyes. He knows the leaning deeply on Jesus, he has walked the moments of utter dependence most of his days, but the quiet reprieve of us vanishing leaves him uncertain. He knows the footing will come, but he dreads the unsure steps of the first moments, first years, first everythings without me. His reaching for me in the morning has become hungry. His counting mirrors my own. Our expressions of love have become special, the small irritations have vanished, our communication has become sweet.

Time is a relentless river. It rages on, a respecter of no one. And this, this is the only way to slow time: When I fully enter time's swift current, enter into the current moment with the weight of all my attention, I slow the torrent with the weight of me all here.

Ann Voskamp, *One Thousand Gifts Devotional*

I have started to talk about life without me. I have been praying for the gentle heart of Jason to know love, walk near to love, and grow in gentleness for our babes, who will be so ill equipped for life without a mama. Our children will not cease to be needy, fussy, disobedient once I'm gone—we know the opposite to be true. Jason's calling will only increase. I'm praying into eternity that the grace for my family will increase. These prayers feel desperate, hopeful, important. I feel as though these future prayers that enter eternity matter. They will meet Jason where I cannot. I will cease, but those prayers will go on and on and on. They will be love that transcends my strength and ability.

I limp along at efforts of quieting and slowing my cancer. I made my pie without sugar, as if that effort would keep cancer away. We know it's worse than that, but it feels good to do something. The stomaching of endless pills feels proactive, and I find myself hopeful in a good outcome, but my hope is not in a cure today. My hope is not in the absence of suffering and comfort returned. My hope is in the presence of the One who promises never to leave or forsake, the One who declares nothing "will be able to separate us from the love of God" (Rom. 8:39). Nothing.

1. Your story is a good story. In the grief, pain, and hard, the Author has a plan. It may feel like a desperate breaking of your very heart, but suffering is not the absence of God or good. In our culture,

the goal often seems to be winning, being the best, most beautiful, most successful, but what if that isn't the good story? How has suffering made your story richer? How has it shaped your story?

2. What about the bitterness of unmet expectations, hopes, and dreams? What have you done with the bitter that meets us all?

3. What specific things have happened to you that have caused you to struggle to be thankful to God? In the midst of your suffering, where did you turn?

4. Have you specifically experienced God's kindness and grace in the midst of difficulty? What faces and actions come to mind?

5. How does your life look different from what you once expected? Are you okay with the differences? Why or why not? How would you describe the new story you are living?

Chapter 4

The Dance Most of All

*... a time to weep, and a time to laugh; a time
to mourn, and a time to dance ...*

Ecclesiastes 3:4

From my littlest years, beauty was always the prize in our house. My parents are beautiful people. I remember watching my mother water-ski, thinking she was simply the most beautiful woman I had ever seen slalom across the water. I loved how she never fell, but would toss the rope high in the air so she could plug her nose as she casually entered the water. She was never a strong swimmer, but she was an excellent skier. Mom was elegant. Elegant in how she spoke, laughed, looked. She wore things like capes and flowing skirts and just the right amount of makeup. At a very young age, she acquired this striking gray streak through the middle of her hair that I've always wanted. My parents always lived large and loved laughter and beauty. Especially beauty. It makes sense: beauty brought them together, attracted them to each other. Attraction cannot be discounted. It does matter; it is often where things start.

But from a very young age, I was a tomboy, stubborn to take hold of the story that beauty wins. Puberty felt like a betrayal when I grew curvy in all the right places. My dad called himself "the hooter king," so proud of the beauties his girls were becoming. I knew men noticed how I looked. I liked it, and it also terrified me. I loved being noticed, and I hated it. I saw the value placed on beauty—especially the busty blonde kind—as false, a lie. Even as a girl, I felt if I pursued beauty, it would lead to an empty existence, one that would know a sad ending. I was angry at my bustiness. It's all I knew, but I wondered if there was more—just something more. I just didn't know how to find it.

I was looking for a way to break the rule that beauty wins. In those years, grunge was what became cool, and I happily hid my features for many years. Pearl Jam came on the scene and gave me a beautiful reason to cover up what society wanted to exploit. I was happy hiding under layer upon layer of my thrift-shop wardrobe. I remember my beautiful mama asking me to buy pants that actually fit and feeling like I had won in some small way when I refused. I was changing the rules of our family's predominant story.

When I first became a Christian, I read Matthew 5:29–30:

> If your right eye causes you to sin, tear it out and throw it away. For it is better that you lose one of your members than that your whole body be thrown into hell. And if your right hand causes you to sin, cut it off and throw it away. For it is better that you lose one of your members than that your whole body go into hell.

As a brand-new believer, I read these verses with fear and trembling. I took my Bible to Jenny Gates, the woman who told me about Jesus, and asked her if this meant I needed to get rid of my large breasts. I'm completely serious. She looked at me utterly bewildered. Then I went on to tell her how men would not meet my eyes but stared at my chest. I told her how I hated how large I was. I broke down telling her story after story of jokes, jeers, and gawks I had witnessed. I couldn't stand it. She calmed my heart, explaining that the lack of self-control in another was not my responsibility, and she had an honest talk about modesty with me.

In my experience, self-hatred is the dominant
malaise crippling Christians
and stifling their growth in the Holy Spirit.
Brennan Manning, *Abba's Child*

It took me a long time to understand that modesty isn't hiding or hating who I was created to be. It has been years of struggling to embrace me and embrace beauty, maybe most especially beauty in the eyes of Jason. I want to live with a beauty that doesn't hide, a beauty that takes into account the unique way I was made, beauty that is not a mistake. This is a journey I am still on today. How do I embrace beauty in a way that glorifies God?

Coming to know Jesus untied many of those knots I had tied myself into in my struggle to figure out how to live in beauty. Jesus knew me, intimately, all of me. He created me, just as I am. But coming to Jesus didn't untie all of them. I still fought against the anger I had from my little years that placed too much value on appearances. I struggled with any notice of my beauty, I cut my long blonde hair, refused feminine clothes, and really became hardened to the way I had been created.

I wanted to be known for more than physical beauty, so I did my best to pursue different kinds of beauty in myself. I became fierce in my hunger for knowledge. I realized in college that I was fairly smart. I also learned I loved to read, and so decided to become an English major. I decided to pursue education because I had a passion to share my new love. I continued to struggle with accepting my body, but other facets of who I was began to unfold, and it was liberating.

Therefore, if anyone is in Christ, he is a new creation.
The old has passed away; behold, the new has come.

2 Corinthians 5:17

I loved that verse, but in my newfound faith, I simply could not imagine what that looked like. I naively thought becoming something new meant denying what once was. I moved from not wanting to be known for how I looked to wanting to be known for my faith. So in those early years of faith, I felt that I was rebelling in a different way—I was running to something healthy. But the truth is, I was still running. I was so ready to live differently that I ran from all that had been a part of my former life. I did not realize that in the rejection of my physical self, I was practicing a form of unthankfulness. Jesus made me beautiful, and He had also made me smart and caring, and they were all tied to one another. To reject one piece of myself would in some way be to reject all the others. In a sense, it was telling God He really didn't know what He was doing.

I remember so distinctly the day I saw Jason that second Colorado summer. I saw him, and he was cute. I did hear him speak and thought he was funny and wise. But first, first I *saw* him. And the same was true for him with me. He *saw* me, and that's where things began; in attraction, in the look. This is something that's hard to write, but it must be said. Our story didn't end there; it was a sweet pause, a comma that caused us to pursue each other beyond appearances. But that's where it began.

What God has patiently taught me over the years is the difference between *pretty* and *beautiful*. Pretty is what was valued in my childhood home, something that involves primping and painting and covering over so as to be acceptable in society's eyes. Beautiful, on the other hand, is the revelation of what is truly and naturally there, often through suffering. This change in my understanding came most dramatically in the birth of our children. Having my children was the most amazing redemption of my body. I felt as though every square inch of the creation that was me was restored through my years of having children. I finally had reason for each of my curves. I could give birth to my babies, and I could nourish them. Nursing was a grace, a joy, the most amazing connection to each of my little faces. It was the place we met every morning and evening and hours upon hours in between. Nursing stopped me, quieted me, sat me down and gave me a special time of connection. Nursing made me stop and pay particular attention to the needs of my babies, to wonder over their faces, to smell their heads, to pray for their hearts. I loved that season of my life, a season that took its toll on my physical body but revealed a beauty I'd longed for since I was a little girl.

Beauty is one of the rare things that do not lead to doubt of God.

Jean Anouilh

Now I am raising three amazing daughters, and it feels like walking the edge of a cliff. Recently I took my daughter Eleanor to dinner to have a discussion about beauty and modesty. She is tall and beautiful, and everyone is noticing the striking *outside* that is developing. But I have seen her heart, and it is such a tremendous gift. We went to dinner and we laughed, giggled, took selfies together, and ate hamburgers. She chose a giant bacon, onion, barbecue something. It was unreal. She devoured it, and evidence of it covered her entire face—it was everywhere. I laughed so hard. I told her what a fun date she would be one day. I told her how in my day, girls tried to act like they didn't eat much food. She was stunned, and she said, "Mom, isn't dating about eating great food?" I love it; that's my Eleanor. No frills, just real, and I think she'll be exactly the same on the date, covered in hamburger, laughing loud with her infectious laugh, and seeking joy.

I talked to her about modesty from a more mature place, from the place of protecting men. Over the years I have come to a more gracious perspective of men. They are visual—wonderfully, visually made. I talked frankly about the differences between men and women, how we may love short skirts and low-cut shirts, but they result in becoming a place where men look. We talked through the gift of her physical beauty, because it is a gift. I told her how I loved the beauty I see in her face, but I talked of the beauty of her heart. She turned to me and said, "Mommy, you know when they say I'm beautiful, I think you should get the compliment, because I'm beautiful because of you. I'm beautiful like you, Mama." I sat in stunned silence at her words. They were a gift. What an incredible contrast to the home in which I grew as a girl. My daughter sees me as beautiful, and in that she sees her own beauty.

Her words were a redemption of my own fear and running, from the fight I have fought for years against the way God made me. These moments raising my girls—Eleanor Grace, Harper Joy, and Story Jane—are the beautiful redemption of my own story. They have known the soft recesses of my beauty as a young mama, and they learned a new depth of beauty as they walked with me through my cancer treatment.

My perspective of beauty was challenged from the outset of my treatment. A lifelong tomboy, I didn't think the losing of my naturally blonde, long hair would matter much to me. After all, I was the one who rarely even remembered to brush my hair. I thought myself impervious to such fuss. I thought my identity wasn't wrapped up in my appearance anymore. I thought my story had already been changed in this area. I was wrong. Or just naive. When I started treatment, I had no idea how bald would meet me. I didn't know how I would embrace it, hate it, walk through it.

Bald. The word itself has no elegance; it's a blunt, matter-of-fact four letters that can refer to a scalp, an animal, even a tire. And that's how I met myself in the mirror exactly sixteen days after the first dose of the healing poison. Early September found my littlest, Story Jane, and me pulling out handfuls of my blonde hair and scattering it to the wind. It was the day my sister, Jonna, flew in, and the day a friend met me in my bathroom to shave my head—*bald.* Without my hair there were the gaunt, deep-set black eyes, completely void of any glimmer, and I was deeply grieved. My weakness showed—no hiding, no faking—just weakness. I hurt at my inability, my bald, my gaunt, my pain. I would love to say I screamed, cried, wept in sorrow. No, chemo brings silence. A deafening silence to just get through each moment. Silence to my robust personality, silence to my children, my friends, my love. Painful, grievous silence where there had once been constant, loving chatter.

Before I met bald, my hair was long, thick, lovely. I hadn't known really how lovely until I lost it all one day. It never returned; it never will. Chemo utterly changed my very DNA. I meet a stranger every day in the mirror. I saw my hip bones that had been buried under years of baby-bearing softness. The soft that met my children in a warm embrace vanished, and I became all corners and harsh. But they still embraced me; they saw it was still me under the veneer of my harsh exterior. They knew my heart; they knew I was there. Thank God. Many days when I passed the mirror, I could not look. I felt like I looked like a giant thumb with big, dark eyes. I remember hearing a young woman say she would be fine if she lost her hair. I quietly sighed, hoping she would never know the pain of the ugly I was facing. I did not admonish her ignorance, only silently prayed she would never have to look for the grace at the end of her day to meet herself in the mirror, utterly changed by chemicals. It's a bottom I don't want another to know, but even at that bottom, there was love. Unbelievable love.

The story that baldness brings is that everyone has entry into your illness without sharing it. I am an outgoing people person, and in my life before cancer I would meet the eyes of strangers with ease and begin a conversation, seeing each conversation as an opportunity to love, to share, to embrace a new person. But bald? When eyes were met, immediately faces were diverted, embarrassed at the looking. Jason noticed I would go out in public with my eyes focused on the ground. When he asked me why, I said it allows people to look without feeling guilty. I felt ugly, and the bald birthed a loneliness in me I had never known in my life. I longed to hear the voice of a daddy tell me I was loved even in that desperate place. I did, but not where I expected to hear it.

As it is those closest to you who can wound the deepest, it is also those closest to you who can love the most profoundly. To have my children kiss my bald head, to have my oldest daughter, Eleanor, encouraging me to brave bald in public, to have Jason pursuing me, even finding me attractive and loving me in that desperate low … this was all something I didn't expect. I learned the heart of beauty in my terrible ugly. I learned a confidence and footing in my life in the unlikely, desperate place of bald and harsh in appearance. And in it all, I heard the voice of my eternal Father accepting me even as He was stripping me. I was becoming more beautiful as I was outwardly diminishing. I didn't expect the new challenge of bald, and I also didn't realize the way I would be seen there, as someone beautiful. But I was.

My dear friend Mickey decided to come in the middle of my treatment and walk alongside our family. She stayed multiple weeks and helped carry us through some very dark days. With each new treatment, I hit a lower low, a weaker weak; the bottom grew deeper and deeper. Mickey came, stayed, nurtured, and protected. She loved us gently in our exhausted state and surrounded the kids in their fearful place with her gentle, joyful brand of love. I remember the first outing Mickey and I braved bald. We went to Costco and lunch. Mickey has a gift for conversation far exceeding my own verbal abilities. We entered the warehouse store talking, and we left talking. I barely noticed the glances and felt utterly free from the uncomfortable wigs and hot scarves. I felt liberated in a new way. We went to a nearby hamburger place for lunch. In the middle of a bite, I found a hair in my burger. Mickey looked at me and frankly said, "Well, we know it isn't yours." We laughed harder than I had laughed in months. It was laughter we needed, exactly when we needed it. Mickey's timing with that one-liner, and also her presence in our home, was right on target.

It is so easy to think we have shed the lies of our little years, embraced a new reality for our story—then we are faced with the practical theology that suffering brings. It shows us what lies we still live with daily. Though I thought I was free of the need to be accepted based on appearances, when faced with the outward reality illness brings, I saw where I struggled to truly believe the goodness of God in my story. God has walked me through the valley of the shadow and shown me what true beauty really is. He showed me what love really looks like, and He built a depth of beauty into my story that a life without suffering would never have known. I never imagined in my wildest dreams that Jason could look on a bald, emaciated, black-eyed, breastless woman and love her. But he has and does. It is beautiful. And humbling.

Il faut souffrir pour être belle.
You must suffer in order to be beautiful.

I desperately hoped chemo and surgery would be the end of my journey with cancer. We had every indication that I had a complete result with my treatment, and I would be free to move on after my bilateral mastectomy. Sadly, though, there was cancer still present in my lymph system. When I went to see the radiologist, he didn't *see* me. He looked right through me and spoke a series of statistics in my face. He told me he was logical; I told him I was emotional. His face finally softened as he saw he was about to lose me in the blur of his numbering my chances. I apologized, saying he had met me as a wearied patient hateful of the scars chemo and a bilateral mastectomy and breast reconstruction had created. He told me I needed more burning rays to extend my days. I went home and wept. The pain after chemo and my multiple surgeries was unbelievable. My pain management was botched in my double mastectomy surgery, and I was exhausted beyond belief of the medical community, especially a community that seemed unable to *see* me.

We opted for forty agonizing treatments of radiation to my upper quadrant. These harrowing treatments came after the chemo, a bilateral mastectomy, and reconstruction. Where chemo was a beautiful gathering of my girlfriends through my darkest suffering, radiation was a lonely island of suffering completely alone. Every morning my dear friend and pastor Carl Nelson would meet me. We would pray, then I would walk the lonesome path to my newest snort. My little body was wearied by treatment and surgery after painful surgery.

The loneliness of radiation is pervasive. In the beginning of my radiation treatments, I was handed a towel as I disrobed. By the end, the ladies, my team of radiation medical experts, were used to my scarred, burned, and painful self. I lost my modesty and fear in front of the kindness of these ladies. Apart from Jason, they were the first I showed my new self to openly. They had seen many Barbie-like women before me left uniquely without nipples from treatment. Over our long treatment together, they saw me, soon learned my story, and saw me. The new me, the broken, beautiful me. These women carefully situated me, lining my body up to the tattoos they placed all over my body. Then like bugs in the daylight, they scattered and left me alone. Painfully alone. Chemo left me with endless days facedown; radiation moved me the opposite direction but equally painful. On the cold table, I was situated and left face up and cold as the snort did its worst, breaking down the rapidly growing cancer cells within my body. This season lasted forty treatments over the span of two months. I was left forever burned, forever changed, and damaged from the inside out. The deep burning we hoped would keep us from future cancer.

When that season of treatment ended, we rang the bell in my treatment center and had a meal of celebration at our favorite French bistro. After that, we packed our bags. We left town for napping, reading, connecting, attempting to forget. All my team of girlfriends were present, family flew in—the works. We shed tears, celebrated, rejoiced. We took pictures, toasted the end of radiation, enjoyed the brief celebration of what we thought was the completion of my treatment.

Groupons for horseback riding purchased, meals planned, travel route designated, a beautiful mountain home donated as well as time at a dude ranch and a borrowed pop-up camper. We were committed to the running away, if only for a little while. We were going to run away and come back forgetting. Together we all conspired to embrace the ending of the horrid year. The doctor assured us of a less than 5 percent chance of recurrence. We bought it, we owned it, and it was our gospel. We had been through the worst, the hardest of everything, and prayed to never return to the horrid reality of the facedown pain of chemo and the face-up burning of radiation. Simple procedures awaited our return, but they weren't pressing. We needed life, living, connection away from the endless appointments and painful living that had been our year.

One last minor surgery remained, and we would get to that later, but now it was time to party, time to forget, time to connect, time to grow back hair, life, energy, and stop our fears of that ferocious disease coming back. I was ready to return to strength. I was ready to move forward. Mostly, my deepest desire was to return weakness back to the place of weakness, and get back to being strong.

But I am not the Author of my story.

> *"I wish it need not have happened in my time," said Frodo.*
> *"So do I," said Gandalf, "and so do all who live to see such*
> *times. But that is not for them to decide. All we have to*
> *decide is what to do with the time that is given us."*
>
> J. R. R. Tolkien, *The Fellowship of the Ring*

I am sitting quietly on the bed of my eldest daughter, Eleanor Grace. I have learned the hard art of waiting on her to share with me. The waiting hurts. She knows how to stall. She knows well how to avoid the tears that need to be shed. But I see the tension growing in her. I have little knowledge how to approach her quiet personality. She needs space, and she needs me to be pushy. It's a tender balance. She carries a weight I cannot understand. She has a knack for holding, withholding, shouldering the heavy burden of now. Her silence is her gift and her sorrow. But I reached the end of my ability to wait. So I asked a few questions, and I realized her grief was so much closer to the surface than I realized. She confessed that she has very few moments without fear of losing me. We both finally let go and spilled our words, shared our hearts, and expressed the burdens weighing us.

The life of a middle-school girl is painful simply by design. My tenderhearted, giant-love-giving firstborn has walked this journey with me, knowing the possible outcome of cancer more than any of the other children. I would catch her listening, watch her eyes grow pained looking at me, and I watched her slowly becoming more quiet.

I pushed, often too hard for her to share her heart. She attempted efforts at *okay* that I never believed, but this wearing journey causes you to question when to push. Finally, one evening we broke, we broke in her bedroom into a thousand carefully kept pieces. It was not pretty, but it was beautiful. Her fear meeting my own of facing future days without me in them. This would be a part of her story. We wept together. I told her how I lacked imagination for words, but I knew God's grace would meet her there. I told her I was fighting to believe the goodness of our story that seemed anything but good.

Too much reality for too tender an age. I cannot change the story, and I'm so ill equipped to protect her from our pain. She admits that she's carrying it for the littlest one of us. She fears for the little attached girl, Story Jane, waking one day without a mama. She feels she has had much of me with her, but she fears the littlest will only have an understanding of my essence. She wept that Story Jane will not get to know me like Eleanor does. Her tender heart was breaking for another, introducing me to a new depth of beauty and love I had not known in her.

I do not know how to protect her from this fear, as it mirrors my own. I'm currently paralyzed by fear, barely functioning. People pray *peace, peace, faith, believe*, but I'm too weak. Too cyclical. Too worn by my story. This week I hear the story of my body, next week the story of my brain. I'm quietly languishing in fear. Not of dying so much, but the fear of when the options for treatment cease. Or the options that seem possible end. The exhausting, most painful, breath-stealing aspect of illness is the constant focus on self. Tests on *me*, results for *me*, appointments to deal with *me*. I'm so weary of my own story I could run away.

Jason recently said in a sermon, "We want suffering to be like pregnancy—we have a season, and it's over, and there is a tidy moral to the story." I've come to sense that isn't what faith is at all. What if there is never an end? What if the story never improves and the tests continue to break our hearts? Is God still good? How does our story of love change when we look head-on at my absence from this life? How do you live realistically when you feel like your moments are fading, fleeting, too momentary? How do you fight for normal in the midst of the crushing daily news of more hard? How do you seek hope without forgetting reality? How do we wrap our children in our love story and continue to live intentionally, getting salty tears in the baked ziti? How do we share the story being written for us with our children while we try to protect their childhood?

Bald can lead to such beauty. But it is never, ever pretty.

1. What is your definition of beauty? Where or who did it come from? Is it serving you well?

2. How do you communicate beauty to your children, especially in a culture that worships only the outward?

3. What about yourself causes you to look downcast at the ground instead of into people's eyes—better yet, instead of into God's eyes? What is the root of that shame? How have you experienced God meeting you there, or wanting to meet you there?

4. What experiences have you been through that have left scars? What are some words you would use to describe those wounds and scars? What are some words you believe God uses to describe your scars?

5. In what ways have you tried to run away from your suffering, pain, hardships? Were you successful? What might it mean to accept your suffering as a vital part of your story, one that could ultimately lead to beauty?

Chapter 5

Shadowlands

… a time to cast away stones, and a time to gather stones together;
a time to embrace, and a time to refrain from embracing …

Ecclesiastes 3:5

It was a Sunday like no other. Jason and I knew we should have asked for help, but the sermon was prepared, so Jason went forward with preaching. We entered the junior high cafeteria, the stark place of worship we meet in every Sunday. The previous week had left us stunned. We were sure the news would be good. We were sure the scan would be clear. We were sure we wouldn't get a somber voice on the other end of the phone line. *Sure.*

What we heard was, "Abnormality. We found an abnormality." And then I was sitting in the audience, listening to my love preach an impossible sermon as his love was sitting in the audience full of new cancer.

That week Jason was preaching on the hard verses in Mark's gospel that cover marriage in heaven, and Jesus's answer that we will not be married in heaven. Since my diagnosis, Jason and I had spent many hours discussing these verses and our struggle to embrace them. These are verses everyone wants to avoid, and I mean everyone. People want to think of marriage existing in heaven and that we all become angels or something and get our angelic wings and then have a say in how the world is run. We know from Scripture that I will never become an angel (please never call me an angel after I'm gone), and we are growing in our understanding that our marriage will end at my death. But we have also embraced the beauty of this hard truth. Painful beauty.

I sat quietly in the audience through the songs with my head on Jason's chest and heaved hard tears with him. The embracing of this truth comes only by a heartbreak. His tears mingled with my hair as he held tightly to me. The worship team struggled through each song, watching the two of us utterly broken in the front row, unable to comprehend if Jason would find the words or if he would simply weep through the sermon.

Jason preaches exegetically, which means verse by verse through a Bible text. He did not choose this week to be the week he preached that we aren't married in heaven. It was exactly planned, and certainly not by Jason. A man we both love says these are the hardest verses in all of Scripture for him to embrace. He sat in the audience that day as Jason struggled for the words to bring life to their meaning.

> And Sadducees came to him, who say that there is no resurrection. And they asked him a question, saying, "Teacher, Moses wrote for us that if a man's brother dies and leaves a wife, but leaves no child, the man must take the widow and raise up offspring for his brother. There were seven brothers; the first took a wife, and when he died left no offspring. And the second took her, and died, leaving no offspring. And the third likewise. And the seven left no offspring. Last of all the woman also died. In the resurrection, when they rise again, whose wife will she be? For the seven had her as wife." Jesus said to them, "Is this not the reason you are wrong, because you know neither the Scriptures nor the power of God? For when they rise from the dead, they neither marry nor are given in marriage, but are like angels in heaven. And as for the dead being raised, have you not read in the book of Moses, in

the passage about the bush, how God spoke to him,
saying, 'I am the God of Abraham, and the God of
Isaac, and the God of Jacob'? He is not God of the
dead, but of the living. You are quite wrong." (Mark
12:18–27)

Jason humbly stood, and the words that came from that sermon
will likely not soon be forgotten. God's perfect timing of having a
man speak on these words in the midst of his own hard of facing
more cancer with me caused the words to sink deeper, the truth to
be more focused, and the grace for this hard passage more present.
He stood before us and opened his hands of the thing he loves most
in this earthly life: *me*. He stood and told us all of the goodness of
God to bring marriage into our lives, a reality to point us to a greater
story. He stood and talked of how we cling to the morsel we have
been fed as a reminder, and forget the banquet that awaits. Then
he broke down and said, "We cling to the shadow *of* the story and
forget the light *in* the story. We love the shadow." He would not let
his eyes meet mine.

Marriage is an illustration, a living illustration of our marriage
to Jesus. Marriage is a reminder, a shadow, a picture of what is to
come. When a marriage is based on Jesus, based on love, on grace,
on the goodness of God in relationship, all who come in contact
with that marriage will go away blessed, richer, nourished. Marriage
is to be the place of freedom to deeply know God's goodness, mercy,
forgiveness, and grace. It is to point us to the ultimate Goodness,
Mercy, Forgiveness, and Grace that is to come. It is the ultimate
"now and not yet" in living.

Our struggle in marriage is holding so tightly to the other and forgetting the picture is the living allegory. At the tender age of forty-two, Jason has been asked to open wide his hands to the picture of Jesus in the marriage he has enjoyed for sixteen years. He had to stand before our church community and confess that he wants the morsel, the shadow, the picture, and the letting go is breaking him in a way he isn't prepared for. He cried through his text, he broke, and he shared from an honest heart. He shared how he struggles with belief, and asked for help in his unbelief through this journey. His words were a bruised grace, the honest grappling with truth we all want to avoid. Many pastors would have skipped the passage altogether and simply let the hard verses sit alone without any teaching, saved for another day. But Jason went through the hard passage, his own clinging, his own desperate fears of our story changing, and pointed to the goodness of God in providing such a picture of grace through our marriage. He stood bravely before our community. He stood bald, with his fists tight, asking for prayers in the letting go. He asked us all what shadows we were holding on to.

Everyone in that room felt the tight grip of life, this life that we cling to. The places we can't see, the graces to come, because we live for the graces that are here. We all had to confess how we see the picture of life as life itself. None of us have the strength to loosen our grip, untie the knots, open wide our hands to the loves we love. We lack imagination for life beyond what we can see, feel, smell, and taste. We are reckless in our grasping for more time, and forget the best is yet to come. We simply have so little imagination for our forever home, and yet I feel that Jesus is very gentle with us in our lack of understanding.

As our story continues to struggle, and the plot of my cancer thickens, God has deepened our love, helped us in our weakness to begin to have an imagination for heaven, and met us in such gentle grace where we cling. I picture God's gentle countenance as I beg for more time, more loving, more enjoying the crumbs, as I can't see the next season in all its fullness. I don't struggle with dying, but I struggle and lose my breath when I think of my family watching me suffer through finding my way to heaven. I struggle as I will see my pain reflected in their faces. I will see their fears in letting me go, and knowing the graces that will follow.

Jason looks upon me with gentleness and longing as I'm offered a new drug, a new treatment, a new short remedy to extend my days. I agree to the pills, the hot flashes, the cutting, the pain, the discomfort, and the struggle to live in the small moment that is now. I struggle for the conclusion, I wrestle with the brokenness, and I pray, oh how I pray, for more days.

We know the conversation is coming, the options will cease, and the cancer will have its way. We have spent hours discussing those moments in our quiet dinners alone. We have learned to talk as tears streak our faces and we speak about our parting days. Initially Jason wrestled with my talking about those future days. He admonished me in my longing to talk. I started from a place of humor, to gently talking through the realities as he could handle the words, the future planning.

The other day I was praying for that woman who might come after me. I prayed God would be gracious with Jason and the kids, and bring them someone who would love them with a fierce uniqueness. I was praying for her to have the grace to enter this place, this hard place of broken hearts with her own special brand of love and gentleness for the hearts of my children and husband. I pray she will be met with warmth and open hearts. And in the struggle against the edges of this life she will face, I pray she is patient.

Jason asked me the other day why I talk to him so much about this next season of his life. He always sits with me in this conversation, uncomfortable at best. I looked at him gently and told him where my heart had changed, dramatically changed throughout my treatment. When I was first diagnosed, I immediately panicked and thought Jason could never love another. No, another woman could never love these children as I love these children. What if she has her own family? She would love them more. What if, what if, what if?

Then, deep into treatment, a gentle tug at my heart came as I watched Jason gently attend to me in the depths of my pain. His love was not from this world. I was shown what a beautiful husband he is, truly better than anyone I have ever met in my life. And then I imagined this place of his heart, his gifting, his giant love in marriage dying with me. I was left quieted by the thought, mostly broken at my own selfishness. The thought of his giftedness in marriage dying with me felt suffocating. How could I rob him of this gift he's been uniquely given? How could I let him look upon his future days alone, with no one to shower his love on in marriage?

So when Jason asked me why I talk about life after me so much in our time alone, I simply answered him with what I know to be true. In the place of my absence, I know my voice will still be alive and well in Jason's head. I know he will wonder on a parenting issue, a church struggle, an edge of life he comes to, and in that place he will hear one of my endless opinions, my endless ramblings, my words, my words, my words echoing through his mind. The conversation between Jason and me will go on past my days—it just will. I have spent too much of this life in conversation with him for the words to stop. So in the place he comes to, wondering if he should try again at the struggle to love, I want him to hear from me. And I want him to hear liberty, grace, hope, and love. I want him to hear permission. I want my words to give him the courage to love again. I want him to hear me say, *You are excellent as a husband. Be a husband again.* I also want him to hear me say, *Be discerning, be cautious, be patient, but don't close your heart to the possibility of love. Go for it, dearest—we met the best of life in the gift of marriage.*

Certainly, I have fears, concerns, anxieties over those future days. Another voice will be entering the house I love with different ideas, opinions, and preferences. I want to open wide my hands to the possibilities that woman would bring to our home, but I certainly have fears. So in those edges, those anxieties, I pray. I pray for her heart, I pray for the hearts of my kids. I pray they would uniquely love this woman and not struggle with a sense of disloyalty to me. I want my children to know I see their dad's great gift at love, and that I want it to continue. But the edges they will face in those moments, I cannot know. So I pray quiet prayers into those moments for everyone.

In the places of Jason's begging for more time, Jesus hears him and loves him exactly in that place and grants me that next breath. But I know, I quietly know, when the time comes for that last breath to take place, a beautiful grace will meet my dear love in that sacred moment. What seems utterly frightening and lonely will be a moment filled with grace and peace. We cannot know it, because that grace has yet to come, but I believe it will be there. I have prayed many desperate prayers for Jesus to be with my loved ones uniquely and unmistakably in that moment. I have prayed for that moment and the moments that will follow. Amen.

Yet, while we are comforted by knowing this, let
us not rest contented with weak faith,
but ask, like the Apostles, to have it increased.
However feeble our faith may be,
if it be real faith in Christ, we shall reach
heaven at last, but shall not honor
our Master much on our pilgrimage, neither
shall we abound in joy and peace.
If, then, you would live to Christ's glory, and be happy in His service,
seek to be filled with the spirit of adoption more and more completely,
till perfect love shall cast out fear.

Charles Spurgeon, *Morning by Morning*

1. Read again those hard verses in Mark's gospel.
2. What things in your life are you clinging to as shadows instead of remembering the light in your story?
3. How often do you think about heaven? If a lot, describe what you think about. If not, think about why not.

4. Who or what would be the hardest thing for you to let go of? If that's a person, why not share that fear with him or her? It could open up a new level of conversation between the two of you.

5. List three "what ifs" you worry about, ask yourself, and struggle to quiet. What lies are you tempted to believe in worrying? What do you imagine God saying to your "what ifs"?

Chapter 6

There, I Said It

*… a time to seek, and a time to lose; a time
to keep, and a time to cast away …*

Ecclesiastes 3:6

It takes courage, humiliating courage, to step aside from your own sovereignty and imagined control and begin looking for the gift that comes unmerited. Yes, I'm talking about *grace*. Grace by my definition is the gift that comes unearned. In a world of unbelievably able bodies, where new diets are fashioned every day to keep my brand of story away, it is hard to realize you may be living in the middle of the best story ever told. That the story of breast cancer could possibly be a good story? A great story even? It would be easier to shake my fist at the test results and scream that this isn't the right story, but to receive—humbly receive—the story no one would ever want, and know there is goodness in the midst of its horror, is not something I could ever do in my own strength. I simply cannot. That receiving comes from the One who received His own suffering for a much greater purpose than my own.

> But because I believe God's plans for me are better than what
> I could plan for myself, rather than run away from the path he
> has set before me, I want to run toward it. I don't want to try to
> change God's mind—his thoughts are perfect. I want to think
> his thoughts. I don't want to change God's timing—his timing
> is perfect. I want the grace to accept his timing. I don't want to
> change God's plan—his plan is perfect. I want to embrace his
> plan and see how he is glorified through it. I want to submit.
>
> Nancy Guthrie, *Holding on to Hope*

Receiving what is before me and fighting to walk in the path that is only lit one step at a time is a daily practice. There are days the truth comes quickly and days the struggle to hear beyond the lies of comfort, security, and health feels impossible. There was a time in the beginning of this journey when I struggled seeing old people. They were what I felt most jealous of in my longings. I remember wanting to ask: *Do you realize the gift you have? Did you appreciate the weddings, the graduations, the moments—all of them? Do you complain about your aches and pains, or do you see the gift of the time you have been given?* It is ugly business to be unkind in your thoughts to the object you most long to become. In the midst of my cancer, I made an idol of time. It was my greatest prayer, my begging pleadings to Jesus: *Let me remain.* In many ways, it is still my prayer, but God has rooted in me a gratitude for my now, my hard, my story, and even my cancer. I still have a long journey of seeking grace that I may never understand, but this journey has taught me so much. Perhaps the humbling, the prying open of my hand to time, and the growing imaginings for my forever tomorrows have become the balm to help me see truth in the midst of pain. The lessons have come, but they haven't come easily.

Cancer is a gift.

There, I said it. I can say that cancer and suffering give the beautiful gift of perspective. It is the gift you never wanted, the gift wrapped in confusion and brokenness and heartbreak. It's the gift that strips all your other ideas of living from you completely. The beautiful, ugly raising to the surface of the importance of each and every moment. I have loved motherhood in all its nuances. I never cared if a baby slept, I enjoyed snuggles, nursed for years instead of months. I have met my kids in the kitchen, on the dance floor, in their bedrooms quiet at night. There were days I loved interacting with my children, and there were certainly days when I wanted to hide alone in my room to consume a book and let my mind think big thoughts. I have loved my calling as a mama—loved it! But to call it simple would be condescending to the calling. It took me years to find contentment in the mundane momentum of loving in motherhood. Before cancer, I sought kindness in motherhood. The days were not all blissful and simple, but life in the midst of little children was never dull. Tiring, yes; boring, no. I begged for grace to point my precious charges to Jesus, but I lived each moment gluttonous. I ate and ate on the joys of parenthood with no thought of it ever coming to an end. I expected a long life; I may have even thought I deserved a long life.

Jason and I would reminisce on the joy of each child. We delighted in each of our four children. We wondered over cowlicks, bright eyes, tiny ears, little fingers, toenails that seemed to point straight up, yawns, sweet sneezes in the sunlight that comes uniquely from the Tippetts. We lived so simply through seminary that we learned the art of joy in the simple moments: teaching a child to pump on the swing, finding joy in digging in the dirt, building a fort with piles of quilts, playing with a cheap flashlight, creating a meal together, and singing really really loud in the car (my joy, not Jason's). We ate up these moments; we thought they would never end. We dreamed of a lifetime of finding the best Mexican food, the greatest farmers' market, the best camping site, building the best fire. When the fateful diagnosis came, we lost our breath. Harper Joy mentioned her special future trip with me. She is my middle child with a fierce and wonderful memory. We were just newly diagnosed and didn't know how far-reaching my cancer was yet; that snort had not been visited. She glided out onto the somber place we were sitting on our back porch and sang the thrill of dreaming about our future trip on her tenth birthday. The trip I had taken with her older sister when she turned ten to speak about adolescence and becoming a young lady. She danced and dreamed before Jason and me. She was eight. Two years felt hard to promise. Through tears she did not notice, Jason and I talked her through that future hope, fighting to join her in hope. We wept that the endless days started to feel limited, and the horizon of my days seemed to be dimming. Harper Joy did not see the sadness behind our smiles—she only saw her mama, her partner in life, her champion, her safe place. She twirled and wondered over the goodness that was to come as we sat silent, uncertain, afraid. She was so lovely in her joy, in her dreaming. I wanted that trip; it became my quiet prayer for the two of us.

Our family had lived as immortal beings, thinking these precious moments would never cease. We lived not knowing their significant importance. The moments cooing over a baby. The painful moments helping a child sound out each new word, seeking literacy. The burned-toast, hysterical disasters of life. Those incredibly mundane ebbs and flows of life, and then you take a mortal blow, a disease that is known for killing, and it brings a suffocating fear.

From the outside, I think people pictured our laughter halting, our joy absent, our hope darkened, but that wasn't the picture we lived behind closed doors. Certainly there were days the journey tried to strangle our joy and made even breathing difficult. But we were always met with the deep reality behind the word *still*: there was still laughter, there was still joy, there were still parties and still celebrations, and even the wonderful experience of Jason's ordination with our growing church community. *Still* is a lifesaving word, a five-lettered fist of hope. And I learned that firsthand in my pain. Time still kept moving, and we were moving in it, but we were changed. Still the days passed, and the kids grew taller, lost teeth, struggled through the bald bottom days with me, but we learned to really see the grace of today.

We still lived in the tension of a full house wrestling with each moment of lunch packing, permission slip signing, sibling fighting, and homework. We savored the new tastes of life with a keen vision for grace. We saw the gifts of skinned knees being kissed, nighttime snuggles, and the endless flow of really dirty clothes traveling the life cycle of the home. Still life passed, but the time, the precious limit on time, helped us see what did and did not matter. We never cared about a spilled drink, but even more now, we didn't care about the appearance of our living. The messy of our life happened before, but our self-conscious noticing stopped. Our jam-stained counters and endless piles of life in corners simply went unnoticed. We paid money to have someone help us manage the living that kept going, but life mattered more than tidy living. Remember, beauty, not pretty.

Give me the courage to stand the pain to get the grace.
Flannery O'Connor, *A Prayer Journal*

Each week I receive emails from people living through and seeking grace in very troubling situations. These broken followers of my story limp along with me, trying to give credit to the generous Giver of peace and keep walking in the struggle of today. Heartbreak upon heartbreak, but the present light of Jesus in the seeking is the essence of all of their stories. There are beautiful stories of courageous humility as they receive suffering and seek grace in the midst of it. There are also stories of those who are being brought low through suffering to show them their beautiful neediness for grace, those heartfelt inquiries from readers who desperately want to know peace.

When I read the countless stories that are sent for only my eyes to see, I learn the power of living courageously broken. I see through the lives of so many facing brokenness they never dreamed and learning again that maybe, just maybe, brokenness is not to be feared but humbly received. Maybe it is our culture that is wrong. No, not maybe. I know it is wrong.

> *"My grace is sufficient for you, for my power is made perfect in weakness." Therefore I will boast all the more gladly of my weaknesses, so that the power of Christ may rest upon me.*
> 2 Corinthians 12:9

The further truth of my story is that cancer has now entered my blood system. Our new reality is a series of doctor appointments and the heavy anxiety of waiting. Once cancer has entered your brain, you win a lifetime of quarterly MRIs. I have met many who have taken that diagnosis and slipped deeply into anger. I understand. It's an easy place to go. But I cannot go there. I have taken a path of seeking grace. It sounds trite putting those words on paper. Perhaps it is. But if God has called me to this hard story, His promise is one of sufficient grace. Sufficient for me, sufficient for my guy, sufficient for my littles.

Before cancer, I waited on the big moments of life while trying to faithfully live through the small. That living feels foreign to me now. I now live in the large, open grace of the small moments and humbly expect the big moments to come. I may be in them, and I may not. My big moments now are not events or milestones, but appointments and treatment. The small moments have become enormous. The fire in the fireplace, the coffee in mugs, the rib tickles, the learning to apply makeup, the singing out loud and off-key— those are the huge moments. Those are the milestones.

For years, I have lived my life openly in front of a lot of young women. I have mentored from a place of permitting my life to be seen—the good, the bad, and the often ugly. Behind our closed doors I tell the story of extending myself to parent in kindness, fighting against shaming and mocking my children. I openly share the ways I love Jason, moving past my own desires and meeting him in his. I share my life, my recipes, my routine in front of anyone interested and teachable. And I share the power of wrong, the ability to not win, and the freedom of repentance and receiving the beautiful gift called forgiveness.

I love sharing from my experience, but in my heart I always longed for the moment to live like this with my own grown children. I long to have different ideas about fashion and debate over how much eyeliner a young lady should wear. I want to feed my kids their fruits and vegetables until the practice is their own. I want to disappoint my kids with my lack of political conviction and passivity. I want to see my kids grow passionate about something—anything—and I want to watch them struggle through the articulation of those passions as I once did, as I still do. I want to be there to pick the wedding dress and help Lake choose the ring for his love. I want to see them as they walk down the aisle with their tender daddy. And I want to see Lake's face when his bride is first revealed to him. I want to see her arrival to him through my tears. I want to see Jason more gray, more wrinkled, more gentled by love and time. I want to see the little legs enter our bed night after night. I want to hear their excuses to keep from going to bed on time: *thirsty, tummy ache, potty, I'm scared, one more snuggle, please—just one more.* I want to wrestle through these beautiful, irritating moments of life. I want to see what my children become, not just in their career choices but in their character. Who is driven, which is tender, who is stubborn and unmoving, who is quiet and contemplative, how my children grow to protect and love one another. The moment the small squabbles stop and deep relationship enters in as it did for Dennis, Jonna, and me. I want to know them. Will they love the mountains as we always have, or will they fly away to exotic places and love the least of these in foreign lands? I want to have them call for my recipes and ask me questions about nursing, loving, discipline, and relationship struggles. I want to irritate them with my lack of practical advice and my asking if they have heard from the Holy Spirit. I want to quietly wrestle in my prayers over their every decision and fight to not give my endless opinions. I want these moments big and small. I want them all.

Cancer has slowed me, caused me to look at my activity and the purpose in it. I look at the precious lives in my home and long to pour my heart into each moment. Sure, I can't share about sex, finances, and dealing with sticky relationships, but I can share my heart, and perhaps one day in my absence, they won't hear my exact words, but they will know the essence of who I am and my heart for their living. Maybe it shouldn't have taken cancer to begin to live this way. Maybe, just maybe, this gift was given to me to begin to look at the loves in my home and seek their hearts in the way I loved those who passed through my home. I still open my home, share my heart, live before whoever wants to watch, but boundaries on my time have been established. Perhaps it should not have taken cancer to create such a space in my life, but that was what it took to change my pace.

Jason and I feel miracles happen around a dinner table. We have loved the grace of a shared meal, and we still see its importance. We have seen the importance of boundaries on our time, but we also see the joy of partnering with our children in love—big family-style dinner love. Certainly, the Holy Spirit works through sermons, books, and conversations, but we see the undeniable power around our dining-room table.

Weekly, we look at our calendar and make sure we meet alone as a family, and we also pray for families that could use encouragement and meet us in this miraculous place of food, questions, and heart sharing. We have seen more hearts changed around a meal than any other place in our lives. We long for this safe place of meeting for our children and for the many in our community who need support and encouragement.

In the early years, I worked so hard to be impressive. My meals were involved, exhausting, delish, and expensive. Jason always found a destroyed kitchen in my wake of loving another, and we often fell into bed absolutely spent in our doing. Fortunately, my heart to please others was revealed in my serving for applause. Certainly, I'm not immune to wanting to be well liked, but the heart of a shared meal is to know a heart, not be the winner of dinner. My cooking now is nutritious, simple, hearty, and simple to clean up or leave until the morning. The heart of our meals is to know the hearts around our table. I had to learn to cast off my longing for approval, to let go of my need to have a meal reciprocated. I had to let go of the perfect home, the matching plates, the flawlessly timed dinner where everything came out hot and lovely. When I let go of having it perfect, I learned the joy of sharing life with the imperfect. When I untied the knots Pinterest and Martha Stewart tied me into, I began to see the joy of together. The meeting of the edges of life around our table. Broken marriages, desperate addiction, unkindness, hard issues with parenting, love, life. Those were the flavors of the meals I remember most—the honest heart sharing, not the perfect roast beef with perfectly appointed root vegetables. No, when all the trying is put aside, the heart has room to share.

There was one Sunday that forever shaped my love of a shared meal. We had invited a couple to lunch, a couple dear to our hearts who had lost their son in a motorcycle accident. Before they came, we prepared the kids by telling them that we were inviting a very broken couple into our home. We told them the tragic story, and how we wanted to move toward their hurting hearts and love them in this simple way by sharing a meal after church. The kids listened and wanted to love them too.

Throughout the lunch, the tenderhearted man wept openly. He very honestly shared the hurt of people distancing themselves from his grief. His wife shared beautiful stories of their beloved son. Every adult at the table was tearful, broken, hurting in the pain of the story. My children were quietly eating their favorite spaghetti made from my favorite friend Autumn's recipe. They were contented eating their favorite meal quietly as hearts were shared. At one point, this broken man met Ella's eyes and apologized for crying. I will never forget her response: "Mama told us what happened to your son and that you both would be here and be sad. I'm so sorry your son died."

In that one beautiful moment, I knew loving people around our dinner table was the right thing to do. Ella knew our heart's desire to love people exactly where they were. She embraced this man in letting him feel safe crying in front of a young family. She could not know the heavy burden of the loss of a child, but her kindness and love were articulated in a way I could not. I thought, *Yes, a child shall lead.*

> *There is no occasion when meals should become*
> *totally unimportant. Meals can be very small*
> *indeed, very inexpensive, short times taken in the*
> *midst of a big push of work, but they should be*
> *always more than just food.*
> Edith Schaeffer, *Hidden Art*

Now we are that family, we are those broken people who need a table to weep at openly. We are the devastated, the lonely, the sometimes lost who need to be reminded of love and grace. We need the safe place to let our tears spill into our soup and spoil our dessert. The invitations exist, the tables are often set for us, but it can be exhausting work to live in the midst of your brokenness all the time. Some days we want to just be normal. I don't want to be a spiritual giant facing a terrible disease. I want to be a mama, a wife, a friend, a member of a community. I get far too much credit for faith when all I'm really doing is sharing my weakness with honesty. I'm not the only one facing these hard moments. I'm just writing about them.

Some days I see my many girlfriends and loves moving toward me, broken and tearful at my latest news, and I want to go back to inappropriate jokes and thrift-store treasures and picking the best shade of gray for my living room. I see those tables set for me, those safe places that want to remind me of Jesus, the goodness of His plan, and the eternity of endless love that awaits me. I see people wanting to be the safe place I have so often wanted to be for another. It makes my heart feel so loved, unworthy, amazed to be graced with such generous love. But at the same time I just really want coffee next to my husband and snuggles with my kids. I don't want to need the safe place; I want to be the safe place once again.

1. Will your children one day look at their little years and feel developed in their musical/sports abilities but not know the essence of your heart shared openly with them? If you answered no, there is *still* time.

2. List five areas of your life where you struggle to give up your perceived sovereignty or control.

3. Good gifts can often become idols in our lives. What have you been given that could easily become an idol? Has it already?

4. Where are you in terms of living vulnerably, inviting others to see the messiness of your kitchen

and your heart? Who could you invite this month to join you in that place?

5. In what ways are you a safe place for other people? Think of someone you know who is hurting. How can you pursue them and become a safe place for their messiness? Not save them necessarily, but be a safe place to fall?

Chapter 7

Faith of a Child

... a time to tear, and a time to sew; a time to
keep silence, and a time to speak ...

Ecclesiastes 3:7

One stark winter morning I woke my oldest daughter to return to the routine of school after a long break at home. I loved the long season of having her and all my babies in my nest, and felt reluctant to return her and the others to the hallways and classes that filled their days. I quietly ushered her through the morning breakfast, teeth brushing, and readiness for a new semester in the darkness of the deep winter morning. She has walked months upon months with me in this terrible beauty that is cancer. She is my quiet one, my listener, my observer. I must look for the treasured moment when her heart opens and is ready to share life and burdens with me. She loves big, she gives herself fully, but she is quiet in the sharing of her burdens. I see them in her face and I know her firstborn heart carries much I cannot understand as I will always be the baby of my family. My own brother and sister, Dennis and Jonna, carry my cancer more heavily than I do.

I long to know the heart of my firstborn, Ella. I ask, I wait, I ask again, and I pray. This morning as she was busily tapping away at her iPod, I asked her if she would read in Proverbs with me. We read through the first chapter and talked through the rich language. Then we were both struck by the last verse.

Whoever listens to me will dwell secure and will
be at ease, without dread of disaster.
Proverbs 1:33

We talked through what this verse really means. When we listen—really listen—to the Lord, looking Him straight in the face, He removes the dread. It does *not* say He removes the disaster. But the *dread* of disaster. Ella and I sat quietly, trying to absorb the meaning of the verse. I wanted to be quiet and listen and not teach or lecture, but this was unbelievably beautiful. If I really sit and listen to God, He will lift the dread. The dread and fear are what so often steal our peace and leave us on the edges of our moments exhausted. We meet the scary of life and forget to turn to God and listen and know His peace. We scramble to control, fix, and protect from hard. The imagined fears and worries often break us more than reality.

With that, I can also take note that sometimes when the dread enters, I'm not doing the hard work of quieting my heart to listen. This is a constant struggle. I'm too often ready with words instead of the needed quiet. I looked in the face of my wise, young daughter and truthfully told her I did not know if or when the disaster of my cancer would return, but I asked Ella to trust with me that in listening to God and knowing Him, He would walk with us and lift the dread. The entering of dread is a new litmus test of my healing. Trust me, moments of dread come. They steal joy, create chaos and fear, and leave me utterly wrung out. Dread exposes my fear and weak faith and failure to trust where my eternal security rests.

We bowed our heads together and asked if Jesus would help us take hold of this new, startling truth. We prayed to live present in the gifts and callings of today without dread of tomorrow. We asked, and we expected, and we trusted that in the knowing and listening, we would find peace and comfort.

Then the Shepherd smiled more comfortingly than ever before, laid both hands on her head and said, "Be strong, yea, be strong and fear not." Then He continued, "Much-Afraid, don't ever allow yourself to

begin trying to picture what it will be like. Believe Me, when you get
to the places which you dread you will find that they are as different
as possible from what you have imagined, just as was the case when
you were actually ascending the precipice. I must warn you that I see
your enemies lurking among the trees ahead, and if you ever let Craven
Fear begin painting a picture on the screen of your imagination, you
will walk with fear and trembling and agony, where no fear is."

Hannah Hurnard, *Hinds' Feet on High Places*

We have had endless amounts of advice and criticism for how we
have walked and talked cancer with our children. Some feared we were
sharing too much; others too little. It's such a fine line that each family must navigate. It has been a balancing act that has kept us utterly
dependent on God for direction. We have stumbled through our hard
days with our children. Just living normally with a house full of young
children is difficult to navigate, but throw in disease, and it feels almost
impossible. It feels foggy, and there is no perfect way to walk alongside
your children through such grievous hard. But we believe the key is
to come alongside them, or they will become angry and fearful in the
unknown. Children are bright and keenly aware of stress and changes
within the home. They will quietly try to overhear conversations that
happen in hushed tones. They know— trust me, they know. We have
walked transparent before our children with the hard of our story, and
we have trusted the Holy Spirit to guide our words and our silence. So
often we are twisted in knots as we await results, and in those moments
we try to remain quiet. We want to give the kids truth, not our fears.

I will never forget the moment I came home tearstained after
hearing the first news of my diagnosis. I found my two littlest, Lake

and Story Jane, dirty and needing a bath after having a busy morning playing with grandparents. They did not notice my tear-streaked
face; they simply were happy to see their mama home beside them.
I quietly ran them a bath and gently washed their soft blonde hair
and wiped their dust-stained faces. They giggled and told me of their
morning playing. In a quiet voice, I told them I would be taking
some medicine and that the silly medicine was going to make me
lose every bit of my hair, maybe even my eyebrows and eyelashes.
They looked at my long blonde hair quietly. Then my youngest,
Story Jane, fell into a fit of giggles. "Mommy, you are going to look
like a boy." And Lake soon followed her in giggles. Not always, but
sometimes fear melts away in a fit of giggles.

One thing that has guided our parenting direction is that we
treat each child as an individual with unique understanding. Our age
range is large. We have older children who understand the weighti-
ness of cancer and others who don't understand the implications of
cancer or death even. We also recognize that we have children with
differing approaches to communicating and processing struggles,
fears, and heartbreak. We have children who will share every emo-
tion and children who want to quietly process alone.

We have walked throughout this journey next to our children.
We've worked and prayed to find opportunities to allow them to
share their fears, their quiet worries, and the pain in the journey. We
have intentionally surrounded our children with a safe community
of friends and families and our new church community. Friends
who look for the moments to love—simply love them in their pain.
Friends who give them a break from hard and provide great belly
laughter and joy. Some fears were closer to the surface and easier to

hear, and some took months to express. We were a community united with the goal to tenderly walk with our children through hard.

The kids witnessed the facedown days. They knew to quietly enter my room, and they learned the art of sneaking in beside me and sharing my warmth. They learned that they were wanted, and though I appeared fragile, I was still me, just quieted by treatment. Lake soon learned to share a love of superheroes in cartoons during my sick days. He would quietly enter, and my face would light up. He navigated my iPad like a boss and found the next episode of *The Avengers*. He would snuggle close and rub the top of my bald head as we watched quietly together. He watched the screen, and I looked at the wonder that was him next to me. The children knew they were always permitted to come close and never kept at a distance, but they were always so gentle, so good at loving me and learning how to catch my love—quiet but sure. When the days of vomit came, we asked friends to keep them from the house. Friends were always on the ready for the moments that were too much, moments when we needed to protect them from the gravity of my struggle. We sought guidance and help in guarding their hearts when it felt too much, even for us. When the bottom of treatment landed me in the hospital, I knew my children were being loved, kept, treasured by our community, our family created through pain. I could rest knowing my children were being loved well.

The school where our children attended partnered with us to love them well. Eleanor Grace, Harper Joy, Lake Edward, and Story Jane were gently loved at Evangelical Christian Academy through the specific hard of our story. Teachers would slow their plans when their tears called for prayer instead of math. The teachers met my children in hard and gently ushered them through each day, meeting the unique needs of their hearts and not focusing on the outward behaviors that often met such hard pain. Each of these teachers had met their own pain with cancer and knew the seeking of grace in the midst of hard. These gifts, these teachers, friends, mothers in our school walked with us. My children were safe to be broken, and in that place they learned beauty anew.

They still expected much of our children and didn't give them a pass on learning, but they tenderly consoled them on hard days. When Eleanor decided she could not focus any longer the last quarter of her year, her teacher reached out to me to help me navigate her weariness and extend her grace. She and Mickey helped me not to be too hard on her, but to gently meet her in her exhaustion at the end of a hard year of struggle.

Mostly, we answered each question as it came, as honestly as we felt was healthy, and we prayed. How we prayed in this season. We prayed for discernment, we prayed for the ability to shepherd their hearts, and we prayed for strength to love them well throughout my seemingly endless treatment. Our church community helped protect the energy I did have for the kids. I would spend the day sleeping so I could spend short moments after school awake. They would enter the home heavy with their school things and meet me in my chair to tell me about their days. When I had the strength and was not on medication, I would drive to pick up the children from school. They loved the normal moments. The moments when I felt like every other mama. We would meet friends on the playground, and I would have the gloriously normal moments of laughter with other mamas after school. Oh, how I longed for normal moments. The kids saw my quiet where I had once been vivacious and full of words and enthusiasm, my deep quiet in fighting to brave each hard moment, but they saw me beside them. Me, right there.

Recently, Jason came in the room in tears and asked me to go and snuggle beside Harper Joy. He was letting her share all her words of her day with him before bed—her favorite time of the day. Then suddenly she turned to Jason and asked, "Is Mama going to die of old age or of cancer?" Jason struggled for the words, but found himself crumpled under his own grief. He came and asked if I could support him in answering. I walked down the hallway and climbed under the covers with my vocal, young daughter. This one longs for the words, to hear the explanations, and process her feelings out loud. She is very much like me. These moments are a gift to my own love of words, feelings, and expressing troubles of my heart.

I snuggled close and she draped herself over me. Her eyes were big and tearful. She wanted to hear from me. She wanted the truth. I knew this was a sacred moment, a moment where the truth was being asked. She wasn't asking for false hope; she wanted me to love her with honesty. I told her I had heard her question, and I asked her my own question in response. I asked her if she believed God would meet her in both of those places. I looked at her face and wondered at her love, her beauty, her tenderness, and I asked her a question many grown people cannot answer or embrace. In the most painful fear and hurts of our lives, will God be good? Not just the simple: God is good, indeed, always good. Not the rote, recited, memorized answers we have been trained to give in the edges of life. But the asking: Is Jesus really good in the awful of cancer, fire, heartbreak, and devastation? In the face of all that is broken, is God good?

I let the tears come that night. I let myself cry before my daughter as I told her I knew without question that the goodness of grace would meet her if I was taken by cancer and not old age. I told her I trusted God with my moments, her moments, and in the midst of our pain. I told her I would always be her mommy, that I was gifted with the joy of doing every day of my life next to her life. That my love would always be next to her, even if I did not get to be. We showered her pillow with our tears, and I went on to name the joys I had in being her mama specifically. I told her the joy of her birth, the wonder of loving her in her infancy. We talked about her little toddler years that were full of wonder and words. How she was always so true and full of love for her big sister. I talked about her quick mind and her easy humor. Then I simply held her and thanked her. I thanked her for getting the amazing opportunity to love her. I thanked her for her tenderness and heart in all that she does. I thanked her that from her birth up to that moment I was given the treasure of loving life beside her. I told her those days have been the fullest and most meaningful I had ever known. Then I asked her to trust with me that both of us have our days exactly numbered in love. I told her my prayers were to remain beside her, but that if the answer isn't yes, to trust God that the story is good.

Her deep blue eyes that she got from her daddy looked at me and agreed. "Goodness will be there, Mommy, I believe with you." We talked about how the tears were beautiful. That though the hard might come and our hearts be broken, that brokenness isn't bad. The tears are evidence of our love for one another. They did not stop that day, and they will not stop in the days to come. But tears are a gift, not something to withhold or bottle up—they are the essence of the best of life. The love here, now, today has grown our hearts, and makes the parting of our hearts suffocating and hard at best. But our tears will be treasured, kept, and stored in heaven.

How do you speak to your young child of grace you struggle to have the imagination to behold? You just do. It's the raw places of faith without sight. It's the painful moments of preaching a sermon to yourself you know you struggle to believe. It's the quiet prayer from Mark: "I believe; help my unbelief." (Mark 9:24). How do you brave the impossible with children? How do you face these heartbreaking moments? You show up. You look at their faces and beg for God to give you His infinite imagination for the goodness of the days to come, the days for which you may not be present. You pray you will be courageous when the hard days come. You pray that, even as the end comes, there will be good days, good moments, that there will still be enough strength for love. You pray for the moments to continue. You pray for the grace in the raw edges to live well, embracing kindness you don't feel. And then you walk back to your room and weep.

Weep that your young child has to lie in bed at night and wonder if they will know their mama in a month, a year, a decade. You weep because you never imagined this would be the good story. You weep because your faith is so weak, but your weak faith is enough when coupled with God's grace.

Trusting God when the miracle does not come, when the urgent prayer gets no answer, when there is only darkness—this is the kind of faith God values perhaps most of all. This is the kind of faith that can be developed and displayed only in the midst

of difficult circumstances. This is the kind of faith that cannot
be shaken because it is the result of having been shaken.

Nancy Guthrie, *Holding on to Hope*

When your daughter wants into the heart of your own desperation, you grasp for the right words, then you leave with a prayer and endless kisses and walk slumped and tearful to your room. Then quietly send a text message to your friend Blythe, who lost her parents suddenly in a car accident, and you ask her to remind you how Jesus loved her in the midst of her loss. She immediately responds with the needed grace reminder. She sends you texts that tell you the grace will be breathtaking. She says your love will carry your little children. She says the story of me will be retold to their little ears, but they won't need it retold, because they will know in the depths of who they are. That the essence of my love will be so present in their lives that they will simply know. I read and reread the text from Blythe and pray for the grace to believe the impossible, and eventually in the wake of endless tears, sleep comes. In the morning, there is toast to be made. The next thing—you keep looking for the next thing until there are no more next things required. And into each next thing you pour as much love as you can manage and hope that love will sustain those you love for a lifetime.

In every season of our lives, we meet the edges of life we never expected. The unexpected pain of life often leaves us only with the choice of how we will endure it. It could be a marriage you didn't expect to break, a job you thought you'd never lose, a difficult child to raise. We all have unexpected hard, but how do we face it?

I was met with an unexpected disease—unexpected in every way. I could never have dreamed the endless appointments sitting on the crinkled paper of doctors' tables and the endless treatment to extend my days. I never expected to be planning my funeral, counting my moments, and fighting for my next breath in my thirties. I never expected to be sitting on my daughter's bed with the sinking feeling her mama was going to die of cancer and not of old age, and not knowing the right words to love her well. Never. But those places, those raw, broken places, are the heart of life. The brokenness of today causes us to look at tomorrow and hope for it. It causes us to ask, "What is it all for?" I could not look with confidence into the face of my young daughter Harper Joy and tell her I would be with her into my old age—that simply doesn't look like my story. No, but I could confidently begin to tell her about heaven.

Behold, I am making all things new.
Revelation 21:5

My imagination of that next place is weak, but my surety of it is not. I do not spend days, moments, hours dreaming of leaving this place for the next, but I know heaven is my destination. I can take my weak yearnings for that place and share them through tears with my daughter. I can console her in our time together and explain how quickly time has passed. I was once a young eight-year-old in the quiet of my bedroom, dreaming of my future. I would look at my door, hoping my mom would come with a glass of water, a kiss, and sing me one more song. Now I'm the mama entering the room of my young daughter. But unlike me, at the young age of eight, my young daughter will begin to dream of heaven—something I never did. She and I will talk about searching for God's grace and naming it in this life and knowing grace in its fullest in the presence of Jesus in the next life. But in the tension between the two worlds, there is mercy for our lack of understanding, our pain in wanting to remain together, our holding on to this place so tightly. All I know is being her mommy. That yearning is who I am. It's my calling, and each moment I live in the grace of that high calling. I cannot divorce myself from my desire to always be the mama and wife to my family—it's how God created me. And my Harper Joy cannot separate her longing to have her mama close and warm; it's all she's ever known. But if the hardest is asked of us, we believe grace will be there.

> *For the Christian, death is not the end of adventure*
> *but a doorway from a world where dreams*
> *and adventures shrink to a world where dreams*
> *and adventures forever expand.*
>
> Wayne Triplett, *Heaven Is Waiting*

One of the highest callings in my life is shepherding the hearts of my children. The rest of my days I get to be a student of my children. I get to learn their hearts, learn the moments when I can meet them best in love—not simply when it's convenient for me. I get to watch, listen, ask questions, and study them. I watch for signs of struggle with life. I carefully ask about their days on the playground, because for a young person that is where their life is lived. I listen for loneliness and pulling away from friends. I look for opportunities to love and *see* my children. And if at the end of the day I haven't had access to the hearts of my children, I grab my giant bottle of lotion and move from room to room and rub the feet of my children before sleep. It is a mother's version of washing the feet of my disciples. I come with my lotion, and I meet each child in the sweet moments before sleep, and my hope is to capture a piece of their hearts. I rub, I ask questions, and I leave behind my prayers for each child.

Since the birth of each of my children, I have prayed a quiet prayer over them for their hearts to know the nearness of Jesus, for their health, for their future husband or wife, and that child's parents as they raise him or her. These simple prayers have been on my lips every evening for years. I then ask for as many kisses as each child's age, then I kiss the bridge of each nose, and the top of each head, and I'm left with the happy smell of childhood. It is my greatest calling to be a learned student of my children. Sometimes my grade is barely passing, sometimes I'm granted grace to see their hearts, and sometimes I'm in a very long season of study before I can understand the heart of my child. It is a joy and sometimes a struggle to keep at the lifetime of learning my job requires. I never feel as though I will be a teacher of parenting, but will remain a student. I cannot share a recipe for parenting, but simply the heart of a student who longs to learn the unique nuances of each of my children.

Stay close, be there, and if the answer isn't yes, trust God that the story is good.

Through cancer, each of my children has struggled in unique ways. When children face seasons of pain or hardship, it comes out in different ways. I would be dubious of a book that prescribed to me how exactly to walk with children through pain and suffering. We stumble through, but we watch and we wait for opportunities to love our children with the love that was granted us.

1. Do you hide your struggles from your children? How do you seek and find the discernment to know how and what and when to share with your children?

2. Think about being a student of your children. How could you spend time today learning their hearts and moving toward them in love? If you struggle to talk about heart issues with your children and focus simply on behavior, ask God for the grace to begin, one day at a time, to pay closer attention to what really matters—their heart.

3. What are your thoughts about heaven? What does it look like? Sound like? Is it a comforting thought to you or something else?

4. What are the last things your children usually hear before they go to sleep? Words of love and affection? Phrases of impatience? Possibly just silence? How could you begin to redeem that special time before they enter sleep each night?

5. When you pray for God to lift you out of fear and dread, do you truly believe He can and will?

Why or why not? What is an example of when He did, and what is an example of when you felt He didn't? How did He show you His goodness in both answers?

Chapter 8

The Hardest Peace

... a time to love, and a time to hate; a time
for war, and a time for peace.

Ecclesiastes 3:8

If I had written a book before cancer, there would have been an essence of themes that would have been similar. Knitted through my writings would have been a familiar tone to what I have written here. Much of this living I have done with conviction in kindness before cancer, but the theme of the importance and meaning in each moment is new. Seeking grace has been a theme since I met Jesus, but it wasn't the very air I breathed to get through each moment—each scary, hard moment. The looking has now become my practice. The naming of the graces, the gifts I don't deserve, is new to me. But I do not believe you need to face cancer to see the value of looking for and naming the graces in your own moments, days, weeks, lifetime. To capture this beauty in your weariness, even if your story doesn't look like mine, will enrich your moments, give you a new perspective, and help you lift your head in the impossibility and pain in living. Hard is hard.

> *Interestingly enough, the most-asked question in the whole Bible—from Genesis to Revelation—is "How long, O Lord, how long?" And the most repeated command from God is "Do not fear" or "Do not be afraid." The people of God consistently cry out for relief, and the God of love bids us trust him.*
> Scotty Smith, *Objects of His Affection*

Cancer has given me the freedom to see my story with me utterly not in it. *Sans Kara.* I saw the grace of care and community when I could not reciprocate my love to the givers. Cancer showed me the beautiful community that could be built into a church that didn't have me doing anything. Cancer showed me the gift and strength of weakness, that in the place of utter inability, Jesus was able. The beauty of the broken was the gift cancer gave to our family. Suffering taught us a new song of what ministry could be. How do I communicate that gift and help you see the love in the lack of expectation without you facing such devastation in your own life? How do I communicate the gift of weakness, neediness, and utter dependence for each moment and the beauty it brought to our community? How do I encourage grace and the freedom to exhale from the endless expectations you place upon yourself?

I can spot myself in so many mamas I come in contact with daily. I see so much going, doing, and wearing out in the effort to find grace. My heart is so full of love for the overachieving mom, and I long to share the heart of slowing and hearing. I see my former self in the mama who is doing every activity, seeking acceptance in her ability, and striving to capture goodness in her going. I recognize the tired eyes and the efforts at speaking with an energy she cannot feel. I want to encourage her to slow down, to rest, to stop—but I know I would not have listened to me. I would have politely smiled and kept moving to the next thing—the endlessness of the next thing. We so often assume we know the Holy Spirit without listening and plow forward in our serving without taking the time to tune in to His guidance.

In heaven everyone and everything is lovable, but as the Lord Jesus said, "If ye love them which love you, what reward have ye?" (Matthew 5:46). In heaven everyone loves everyone else, and in hell no one loves anyone. But on earth we are in a perfect environment for learning how to love as God loves: to abandon

> *ourselves to loving apparently unlovely people who remind us*
> *that in many ways we are still very unlovely ourselves.*
>
> Hannanh Hurnard, *Hinds' Feet on High Places*

I could not see the horizon of heaven before. I knew it was there, but I didn't believe it was anywhere in my near future. I had planned my story. Old age, really old age, with old Jason. We were doing marriage well, the best I had ever seen it done. In my arrogance, in my pride, in my invincibility, I never imagined the most beautiful story for my love, my life, my kids, my community would be the placing of my mortality in this life right in front of my face.

Last night Eleanor joined me in the making of biscuits and gravy. We wanted to surprise Harper Joy with her favorite dinner. I wanted the moment to teach my daughter as my grandma hero Elnora Lakes had taught me. Eleanor was next to me stirring, beautifully present at my side, when a song we love began playing. We questioned if we could step away from the watched sauce. We decided we didn't care if the gravy scorched—it just didn't matter. So we danced like old lovers. I held her hand in one of mine and her small twelve-year-old waist in the other. She rested her head on my shoulder, and we danced. We danced as Stevie Wonder sang his heart out in "You Are the Sunshine of My Life." I held her through the sweet love coming from the speaker: *You are the sunshine of my life, that's why I'll always be around.* I silently cry the words, because I know I cannot fulfill the promises of the song. Perhaps my body won't be there, but my love certainly will.

We dance and we hope and we know quietly that my love will always be around, even though this dance may come to an end. We ended in a hug, then we silently returned to our stirring. My eyeballs were sweating in my relentless desire for the moment to never end, for something to remain.

> *We danced to the old music,*
> *convinced we have nothing,*
> *really. Nothing but ourselves.*
> *Ours was not a dance of steps*
> *but rather containment, a*
> *dancing in place.*
> *We danced in the arc of*
> *memory, safe, swaying to*
> *the dream of both men*
> *and angels, the only dream*
> *really: that something may*
> *remain.*
> John Blase

In the small town east of Indianapolis, where my grandparents' farm was, there is a little nursing home where the heroes of my childhood now reside. Their farm has long since been sold—that land of the singing cicadas, fireflies, and fishing poles now holds the memories of another family. Grandma sits slumped and silent in a chair day after day. When I first had my diagnosis and we didn't know my prognosis, I turned to Jason and said, "Grandma always looked for my arrival. What if this time, I'm the one looking, and I get to greet her with love and warmth in heaven? Wouldn't that be such a surprise?" Jason and I quietly cried in the car. All my treatment has made traveling to sit beside her silence impossible, and I desperately miss my grandma and grandpa. Had Grandma known what I was going through, she would have walked to be by my side. She would have found a tea set and fancy hats to play endlessly with my girls. She would have found guns to play cowboys and Indians with Lake, and she would have never left.

Tonight my son, Lake, wondered at my hair returning. He asked me about chemo and my heart in the battle. It was a gift of love hearing him tenderly speak to me and reach out to my heart, wanting to know my journey. We then bowed our heads and thanked Jesus for the return of my hair and the break from chemo. Lake asked Jesus that I wouldn't have to return to the place of bald, quiet, sick. Lake always prays for chemo to never return. To him, chemo was the devastating piece for me—not the medicine. I understand. Cancer has never made me sick, but chemo, well chemo is a brand of sick all its own. It was such a grace to see gentleness grow in his heart. If I fail to slow down to listen and look for the graces in the busyness of life, I won't see this develop-ing story of mercy in my son—the tenderness and sensitivity that have grown through our story of suffering is beautiful.

I have confidence of my next life, but my vision of it is dim when I look upon the faces of my little ones. It's a gift and a chal-lenge, living in the now and not in the fear of what is to come. I have no fear of death; I only fear seeing the effects of my suffering in the faces of my loves. Their struggle in the parting. I know my destination; I know I will be met with goodness and my ultimate life in God's grace. When we moved to Colorado and Lake entered preschool, in a short time his lead teacher stepped back from her leadership in the classroom. I did not know at the time, but she was dying of melanoma. I remembered after she was gone to heaven, Lake turned to me in the car and said, "Mama, heaven is so much better than this place. Mrs. Doane is there, and I will meet her one day." I often hear Lake telling others in passing how much better heaven is going to be. Sometimes I feel he is more sure of heaven and hope than I am. It's as if he simply knows. It has been decided for Lake, and from a young age he has a beautiful longing for his forever home. I pray for the grace to have his faith, his peace in leaving, and his strength of love to let me go—knowing my final destination.

> *The sweetest thing in all my life has been the*
> *longing—to reach the Mountain, to find the*
> *place where all the beauty came from ... my country, the*
> *place where I ought to have been born. Do you think it all*
> *meant nothing, all the longing? The longing for home? For*
> *indeed it now feels not like going, but like going back.*
>
> C. S. Lewis, *Till We Have Faces*

"Dear heart, the purpose of life is not longevity."

That's what a friend said to me recently. The words slowly seeped into my soul. I digested them gradually. I hate them, and I love them. I remember the Westminster Confession that asks one simple question: "What is the chief end of man?" The answer, the beautiful answer every heart needs to hear: "To glorify God and enjoy him FOREVER." That *forever* being this side of heaven and the next. Longevity is not the answer, but it is my soft heart's desire. But to give glory forever—yes, yes. That is my longevity in this place and in the next. It is easy to say those words when things are bright, but when future days feel like they are dimming, it's hard. It's just so hard.

> *God's purposes in present grief may not be fully known in a week, in a year, or even in this lifetime. Indeed, some of God's purposes will not even be known when believers die and go to be with the Lord. Some will only be discovered at the day of final judgement when the Lord reveals the secrets of all hearts and commends with special honour those who trusted him in hardship even though they could not see the reason for it: they trusted him simply because he was their God and they knew him to be worthy of trust. It is in times when the reason for hardship cannot be seen that trust in God alone seems to be most pure and precious in his sight. Such faith he will not forget, but will store up as a jewel of great value and beauty to be displayed and delighted in on the day of judgment.*
>
> Wayne Grudem, *The First Epistle of Peter*

The veil between here and heaven is very thin. But it's a dreadfully painful one. We struggle to see beyond these days and look upon eternity with gladness. God gives us morsels of eternity over here, crumbs really, and we beg for them to remain when there is a feast awaiting us. We beg for scraps when the very best is promised. I look at the beautiful creations of my loved ones and say, "Jesus, You did so well—so wondrously well—can't I stay a minute longer?"

I beg for that, really. But His peace answers my heart that it's exactly decided and it's beautiful. It's nothing to be feared. That it is amazing, the story that remains on this side of the veil and the one that awaits on the other. But I need reminding—constant reminding. This, for me, is the hardest peace. I need truth tellers all around me to speak the goodness of grace that will meet me on both sides of the tender veil.

They shall hunger no more, neither thirst anymore;
the sun shall not strike them,
nor any scorching heat.
For the Lamb in the midst of the throne will be their shepherd,
and he will guide them to springs of living water,
and God will wipe away every tear from their eyes.
Revelation 7:16–17

There was a day Jason and I took a shower together. I was bald and done showering in one second, but I stood next to him and heard his broken heart speaking of heaven. He looked at me through tears and shared his heavy burden. He simply said, "Kara, you will be in the land of no more tears; you will not miss me, but I will be here missing you."

I could not breathe at his pain; I could not make it better. I knew he was right. But I also believe a unique grace will meet him in that loneliness that we don't know about yet. It's the chapter I want to write but don't get to today. The story of the breathtaking grace that will meet my loves when I'm gone. But I know it will be true; he knows it will be true. We don't completely understand this, but we still love.

Each one of us here today will at one time in our lives look upon
a loved one who is in need and ask the same question: We are
willing to help, Lord, but what, if anything, is needed? For it is
true we can seldom help those closest to us. Either we don't know
what part of ourselves to give or, more often than not, the part
we have to give is not wanted. And so it is those we live with
and should know who elude us. But we can still love them—we
can love completely without complete understanding.

Norman Maclean, *A River Runs Through It and Other Stories*

My dad recently came to my house for Thanksgiving, and upon leaving he quietly admonished each of my children to be good for Mommy and Daddy, that we needed them *to be good.* I winced in pain. I wanted to scream out at the lie of living to perform. The lie that good acting, good performing, good behavior is what Jason and I need to get through our hard. I respectfully kept my mouth closed (a minor miracle). It was this moment of understanding my dad that made me both love him and feel so sad for him. In the absence of grace, there is only right and wrong, black and white, and the endless unknowable gray of performance. It's true, well-behaved children would help in the moment, but would I know their hearts? They could perform great acts of perfect behavior, but what if the greatest act of theirs now is messy, painful, and not tidy? That is what our story is now.

I understood in that moment the tension my dad has lived under for so many years, and those moments of stress, those painful moments of anger during my childhood were his own inability to fix something. Now he cannot fix what is broken in me, and that must be so desperately painful. So he stumbles through the darkness of today and attempts to help. It's beautiful, really, and I'm so bad at receiving it, because we want love the way we give it, not the way it's given. His rough edges have made my receiving his love difficult at best. I struggle to meet my dad in love when his answers, his fixing, his loving no longer reflect my own. My edges are revealed and they don't draw in my dad, who is struggling with his own brokenness, but they keep him at the distance he has placed himself in: lonely and far off from my story. He's my dad—of course he wants a different story for me. But he is not the Author of my story.

Yes, as the writer of Ecclesiastes says, there is "a time to keep silence." But now is my time to speak. Grace is worth the effort. Grace is worth the hurt, the naming, the wondering at every single day. Grace is the gift of love I cannot earn; yet every day I swim in from hard snort to hard snort. Grace is what meets me after I run to the bathroom to be sick when I think on my reality. Grace is what will meet my children when I'm not here. I don't know how, but I know it will. Grace is the sweet moment you never expect but turns up to get you through a day, an appointment, a reality you never, ever dreamed for yourself.

Jesus didn't have to extend His love. He didn't have to think of me when He went up on that cross. He didn't have to rewrite my story from one of beauty to one of brokenness and create a whole new brand of beauty. He simply didn't have to do it, but He did. He bought me. He bought me that day He died, and He showed His power when He overcame death and rose from the grave. He overcame my death in that moment. He overcame my fear of death in that unbelievable, beautiful moment, and the fruit of that death, that resurrection, and that stunning grace is peace. It is the hardest peace, because it is brutal. Horribly brutal and ugly, and we want to look away, but it is the greatest, greatest story that ever was. And it was, and it is. It is not some storybook pretend tale we read to feel better about today. It happened; it was painful; my sin put Him there, but His love saw me, looked on me—on my heart—and said, *She is Mine. She is My daughter. I have something wonderful for Kara, and it's going to be hard. She will struggle to see Me, but I'm always, always there. She struggles to see Me there for the future of her children and her love, but I'm there. She can't see around the fog of her own pain for her parents, but I'm there. She sees all that is broken, and I see all that is beautiful.*

Grace; it's all grace. Jesus will be there; He will be wooing, loving, meeting my love, my babies, my community, my family, and you long past the day my words run out that beg you to look for grace—that long for you to know Jesus. Really know His love. It's His story, not mine. It's His grace extended, not mine. I have only been a steward of that grace, a simple namer of His unbelievably reckless love that shows up for one broken woman every single day.

I was given the grace in that small moment to not dishonor the heart of what my dad was trying to do in asking my kids to behave. His intention was to be helpful, but what that moment revealed was the heart of one who is facing a brokenness I do not know. I cannot imagine the pain of a parent seeing the suffering of a daughter. I cannot. I do not think I would want to look upon that suffering if I didn't know the answer and gift of grace. So in those edges, those painful places, my dad and I do not understand each other. But there is grace. Grace extended. Grace received. In the places my parents, my family, my community cannot fix, there is grace. Later, in brokenness, I expressed the truth I now know to my children. Living—the living of today—no matter the circumstance, is painful. It hurts deeply, relationships are confusing, obedience is unknowable at times, and the right path is hard to come by some days. But their disobedience does not disappoint this mama. I do not have the expectation of goodness for my children. That is not the truth of the gospel, not the truth of grace to a hurting heart. The truth is, there is only love. Only love.

I write these words without the strength of knowing if I will one day see these pages bound. Since the beginning of the writing of these pages, cancer has returned yet again—this time to the lymph system surrounding my heart. I write the raw edges of my previous days, my current days, and my days to come and feel the moments fading. But for today, this day, it is here before me as the gift it truly is.

> *So take seriously the story that God has given you*
> *to live. It's time to read your own life, because your*
> *story is the one that could set us all ablaze.*
> Dan Allender, *To Be Told*

1. What masks have you worn that have been peeled off through suffering? How did they come off, and how did you respond? Have you been tempted to put these masks back on?

2. At what points in your life have you been given a clear perspective to view your story as part of God's greater and bigger story? How did this impact you and how you live life now?

3. Are you suffocating under expectations you've placed on yourself? What does God say about those expectations? What does freedom in Christ look like in light of these expectations?

4. What plans have you made that have not or will not come to fruition? What has processing your disappointment been like? What would it look like to trust God with your disappointment?

5. Imagine God speaking to you, pointing out moments of grace in your life. What would He show you?

Letters from Kara

Dearest Jason,

   Bright Eyes wrote a song "First Day of My Life" that says, "This is the first day of my life, I'm glad I didn't die before I met you." When I first heard these words, I wept. I feel like life—the life I've hunted for as that little, broken girl sitting beside the river—started with you. I'm so grateful for each moment, each breath, each giggle, each moment next to you—a lifetime of knowing the big and small places of each other. Together we have built a lifetime of living, embracing, laughing to stomach each moment. Always laughing. You know every corner of my heart—ugly and beautiful. You embrace each morsel of this messy me, and meet me with grace and generosity. You give me the courage to over-share it all—on my blog, in these pages, with friends—because at the end of the oversharing, I'm loved. All of me. Loved. I never fret a mistake. I never fear you moving toward distance. You have spent your breaths, your moments, your love moving near to my heart. You remind me of goodness when the story begins to suffocate. The one moment next to you was worth all that has been painful. You have given me moments of grace when I placed you in the place of Jesus, but you always shepherded me back to my true love. Always reminded me of my true heart, the answer to my deepest need. Jesus. You have led me so gently and so well.

   While cleaning—let's be honest, while looking for a reason to not clean today—I found the journal I started for us so many years ago. The journal where we were going to write down the dreams we had for our marriage and our life together. I wrote only three entries in it. Sounds like me, all ideas and little follow-through, but I like to imagine I put that journal down and walked into the beautiful horizon of our marriage and stopped trying to create idols of what life should look like, and actually just sought life and faithfulness in the living. I'm sure in some ways we did that, in some ways we didn't. I will share two of the dreams I listed all those years ago when we were babies trying to figure out how to love each other well.

My first dream for us is that our love would be unceasing. That we would both give to each other in the motivation to see the other grow. My hope is that our love would be enriched as we get to know each other better. That the passion we have for each other would be intensified rather than dulled.

The next dream is to have children. Everything in me knows that I am made to be a mother. All that I do now is to prepare a healthy environment for my children to be raised in. My dream is not only to have children, but also to be a wonderful mother who displays unconditional love to my children.

In so many ways, we met these simple and huge dreams, exceeded these dreams, met our limitations in these dreams, and found this life of ours. Stumbling next to you has always promised to be a safe place to fall. You have walked in grace before me, whispering truth, reminding me of love, giving me freedom to walk, run, stumble, and fall in the confines of your loving acceptance. A love I had not known in another person before meeting you, you have given me an environment to flourish within. You have given me the motherhood I longed to have. You have blessed me with your kindness in the face of unkindness. You have gently led me, loved me, protected me, and shown me a true Jesus. Not the Jesus I want to create—easy, comfortable. But the real Jesus who takes love seriously. A Jesus of mercy, truth, grace. You have faithfully walked your faith before me.

Dear heart, you do marriage so well. Pridefully, I think it could be one of the greatest accomplishments of your life. When I was first diagnosed, I hurt at the thought of leaving you, possibly sharing you with another. Then one beautiful day it dawned on me. Would I really want this man who does marriage better than any I have ever met or seen— would I really want him to give up that beautiful place in his heart, in his life? As you often have seen, Jesus is patient and kind to point out my selfishness and pride.

Dearest husband, you have done husband well. You have loved me so big; you have loved me so wide and so deep. Jason, if I said it all day every day, in my dreaming, in my waking, in my loving, in my arguing, in my writing—Thank you and I love you—it wouldn't be enough. You gave me the life I never dreamed possible. You have braved your faith with integrity in front of this pitiful, weak vessel, and it was beautiful to behold. Beautiful to be led by such grace.

Keep loving big in your servant-hearted ways. Love with gentleness, especially when the gentleness is hard to come by. Give it away; there is no reason to keep it to yourself. I know your heart is about to break into a million tiny pieces. I believe something beautiful is going to grow out of that terrible, ugly hard. I'm afraid, but I'm not afraid for you. You will wake to the daily faithfulness you have walked in for years through hard upon hard. The plan is good, even if the path is hard. I trust Him, I trust Him, I trust Him!

My Dearest Littles,

Oh how I wish this letter were written to my grown children. How I yearn and pray for long days with each of you. Sometimes I see glimpses into what you each are going to become, but there is so much of your story not yet written. As any mama would desire, I want your story to be a beautiful story. I have always longed for a beautiful story where each of you learns to lean into Jesus, love Jesus, know Jesus, understand that His nearness is your good. I never imagined that beauty being accomplished in hard—suffocating hard.

Reflecting on my own heart, my own growth, my own embracing of truth, it came through deep hard, desperate hurt, and brokenness. I know, that I know, that I know, that this was how God grew beauty in me, but I quietly longed for your story to be different. I hoped the deep love your dad and I share and have for each of you would be enough to make your story amazing. It does, but ugly beautiful is part of your story as well. I pray your hearts do not grow hard, bitter, or angry at the hard that has entered your life.

I want to be there. I want to see who you become, how God shapes you. I want to see if you choose lots of makeup or none. I want to know if you love to hike or prefer to snuggle to a book. I want to know if you fiercely enter community expecting the best of life or if you quietly observe and receive love in small graces. I want to know how you smell. I know your baby smell; will that follow you or will you join me in wearing hippy essential oils? Will you remember in tastes and scents of moments? I want the moment when all of you children gather and confess the sneaky things of childhood Daddy and I didn't see, didn't know. The sibling secrets confessed in the safety of adulthood. Places you hid the food you didn't want to eat or the trouble you found when we were away to dinner. I want the laughter of the moments confessed and forgiven. I want the moments when you tell me of my failures and the times I hurt your heart. I want to be there to enjoy the beauty of reconciliation in my weakness and repent of my sin and hurt I inflicted on your heart. I want those moments. I want to ask your forgiveness and learn a new love in the place of our forgiveness.

I want to know your loves. I want to walk through the hurt of your loves big and small. I want to always be the comforter who points you to the Comforter. I want to know you, really know you. I want to ask hard questions and be asked hard questions in return. I want to be with each of you when you reach the age of understanding and remember this hard season with cancer. I want to hear how we protected you, how we failed, how we showed you grace. I want to process the returned pain of your memory of your sick mama and hurting daddy. We loved, we loved, we loved, but we keenly knew the weakness of ourselves in that season. I want to be with you as you begin to process that season fresh as an adult.

I want to dance. I want to dance at your graduation, your wedding, while we wash dishes, when days are painful. I want to dance to loud music, quiet music, music that reminds us of our limits. I want to slow dance with you on my toes, fast dance silly, and just dance because it's Tuesday.

I long for the want of these moments to make them so. As I have breath today, I will live the life I have been given to love as well as I can. I will seek forgiveness in my failing. Each breath is a gift, as each of you children has been to me. Past Jesus and your daddy, you are the very richest gifts. You have shown me love I didn't know I could feel. You introduced me to limits in myself I did not know. You all showed me to seek grace at the end of myself. You have extended sweet forgiveness when I flew from the boundaries of grace and kindness. You met me in my bottom with love and laughter. You walked our hard with beautiful grace.

The hardest part for me is ending this letter. I never want it to end. I want these words, these loves shared, these graces to never stop being named. I want to sit around every meal, hearing the intricacies of your days. I want to put the meal before you but feast on your living, your loving, and your hard. So as long as I have breath to breathe, I pray my living will be a naming of that goodness. I pray you learn the naming long past my last breath.

Eleanor Grace, Harper Joy Sonnet, Lake Edward, and Story Jane: I love you. I love being your mama. I love each moment I was granted beside you. When you meet the edges of life, the hard moments, the suffocating realities, I pray you would look to Jesus. I pray you would know His goodness, and in those edges know my prayers are meeting you—uniquely meeting you, even if I cannot. Thank you; thank you for all you have taught me of life. What a gift each of you is to my heart.

Letter from Jason

There is an older couple, maybe in their early seventies, who regularly walk in our neighborhood. Always next to each other. In the summer, they hold hands, but so far never in the winter. Sometimes I overhear words they exchange, but I can never understand what they are talking about. Grandkids maybe? Kids? A long retirement together? Our assumptions of people are many times mysterious.

As I write this, Kara and I are awaiting the results of another PET scan; this is beginning to settle in as our pattern. I wait, and my mind goes all over the place as I ponder our mysterious future. How will this test that I can't explain change my future, my next hours, days, months and, yes, years?

I think about the older couple often because they hold something that I want. Though I have no idea what they face, I imagine theirs as a pleasant life. Pleasant enough that they don't hold hands in winter. Truthfully, I have avoided meeting them. They hold the picture of what I want.

I know a man, who I rarely talk to but I would call a friend, who embodies the opposite. He has walked the path of losing a young wife to cancer. I avoid him, though I know the day is coming when I will call him and all I will do is cry. Because a mystery will be gone. The unknown will be less mysterious. The imagined dark days will be known.

It is the mystery of life that I hate, the unknown, the confusion, the truth that I am powerless against what I fear the most. As you have just finished reading Kara's words, you know she deals with the same—living in peace when life screams something different. Even though our path carries a story of cancer, I would never trade a day that Kara and I have shared together. Never.

All of us know something of the mystery of this life. As you have read these words, I hope that you will move toward the One who knows the mystery and has a purpose for all things. I hope your deep questions will be answered by the grace that is present, that you will know family and friends and community, and that you will understand a peace that runs through this world and beyond. I am a witness that it is hard, but it is beautiful.

Acknowledgments

I need to start by saying this section has kept me up nights. I'm an extroverted embracer of people who feels the limit of her days. I struggle with the thought of leaving someone out in these next lines—I'm such an includer. There are simply not enough pages to capture all the people whom I have loved, who have loved our family, and who have made an impact on our life and faith. I will feebly attempt to name the countless faces that have met us in our journey, but you are here—so here in these lines, even if I forgot to acknowledge your love. Your hearts, your love, your life lived next to mine is a gift to me. I'm endlessly thankful for all the people who have been a part of my life, enriched my story, and took the time to share my heart.

To the entire team at David C Cook, and specifically my editor, John Blase, who gently encouraged this book out of me. John, you have been a gift of kindness and care to our family by helping us share our story. You are the best kind of poet—the kind who sees the treasure in each moment. You brought your poetry and life to these pages with me, and I'm indebted forever. Ingrid Beck, Amy Konyndyk, Ginia Hairston Croker, Alex Field, and Don Pape—your support behind this book and your encouragement of my voice have been a gift to my heart, a redemption of my story, and a voice and face given to this terrible disease. When October comes and everything turns pink—know you were a part of giving a face to all that pink. Thank you.

To my parents: Dennis and Carolyn Thewlies, Ed and Lynn Tippetts, and Sharon Kirk, thank you for loving us. My sister and brother, Jonna McMahon and Dennis Thewlies—the ones who know it all, hear it all, and know how to bring laughter to my broken heart: I love you. I'm so thankful I do not have a memory in my childhood without each of you next to me. It's good to be the baby of the two of you. My siblings in love and marriage: Mike McMahon, Angela and Dana Weaver, Krista and Josh Grant—love, you all bring such love and care. It was a great good day when we became family. To my grandparents, Homer and Elnora Lakes, who hold the laughter of my childhood—how I miss you. My grandma in marriage, who has been my champion in every way, Martha Tippetts, and her spectacular daughters, Clarice and Annie, who rally me with their prayers—thank you. My own aunt Jan, who loves me big.

My many mothers, mentors, loves—you have taught me the best of life, the embracing of today, and the joys found in simple living and loving my people and walking near to Jesus. Thank you for sharing faith, life, and joy. Vicki Mauro, Jenny Fitzgerald, Mickey Gauen, Sharon Pummel, Shaunda McQueeny, Ruth Durgin, Mindy Belz, Lois Greenlee, Darnell Dietrich, Susan Jett, Juanita Lonon, Julie Eargle, Polly Petro: thank you for always keeping the coffee ready and the conversation and love plentiful.

To my girlfriends: Life with girlfriends is the life I love to live. You all remind me of the best of life, and I simply could not survive without you next to me. From my littlest years until this very moment, my friends have helped me live well, walk through hard, and learn the best of today. This is the place I struggle; I love you all so much, the thought of forgetting a single one of your hearts fills me with dread. Dear ladies, I love you, and you have been the grace, the beautiful grace in my suffering. I know you will walk with my littles beyond my days and remind them of Jesus. I trust you to remind my people of goodness, grace, and the great love I lived next to each of my littles. I love you: Courtney Young, Amy Larsen, Chantelle Howell, Lisa Garland, Kristy Kennedy, Kara Betts, Anika Colvin, Anna Iervolino, Sarah Ritzmann, Jess Bridges, Debbie Richards, Brenda Watt, Trisha Swart, Alison Abel, Liz Corson, Amie Adams, Lisa Anderson, Justine Atkins, Chris Rapert. My ECA mamas—each of you. My playground mamas, who greet me with kindness and care, my classroom partners—my laughter, my love—I love you all, each of you: Erika Counts, Heather Morgan, Corrie McClure, Amy Albright, Connie Russo, Allesandra Hightower, Cathy Dawson, Laura Wilson, Amber Scott, Tracie Biles—this list could go on and on … thank you … The love of you mamas is giant, amazing, important. Love to one another and love to your littles.

To the couples who have loved us, lived with us, and pointed us to Jesus: Derek and Angie Strickler, Bobby and Shari Underwood, Craig and Megan Dunham, Julianne and Joel Adams, Chris and Brandy Baker, Troy and Susanne Rowe, Lori and Philip Sealy, Skip and Autumn Stanley, Mark and Mary Schumann, Jerry and Darnell Dietrich, Lois and Kenny Greenlee, Tom and Marcia Lewis, Sibyl and Bruce Byrd, Nichole and Chad Toney, Tracey and Eric Adkins, Mark and Jen Whipple, Jeff and Troy Hutchinson, Jonathan and Sonja Inman, Donnie and Kara Williams, Calvin and Susan Jett, Tina and Mike VanAresdale, Jennifer and Jacob Stuart, Kerry and Kirk Singleton, John and Thea Kim, Jeremy and Diane Reeves, Mandy and Larry Wilkes, Kit and Karl Wilock, Susan and Jesse Gosner, Rod and Libby Vansolkema, Tim and Jennifer Ayers, Michele and Tom Prible, Douglas and Jody Hammerstrom, Leigh and Jason Davidson, Terry and Jill Buteyn, Cristy and Jim Ross, Lisa and Chris Hooper, Bill and Sue Tell, Doug and Nicole Tharp, Jim and Pam Alexander,

EJ and Joan Nusbaum, Jorie and Steve Roth, Don and Mona Tharp, Lee and Betsy Benson, Jonathan and Aimee Kuiper, Caitlin and Pete Matthews, Stephanie and PJ Mendicki.

To Village 7—elders, pastors, friends, community—you have loved our family so well. Mark and Tricia Bates, you have been our champions, our supporters, the safe place for us to be broken. Mark, you always remind us of truth and point us to the trustworthy sovereignty of Jesus. Carl Nelson, my prayer, my neighbor in treatment, my reminder of goodness, I could not have stomached many of those hard days if I didn't know you would be there waiting to remind me of Jesus.

Sharon and Matt Morginsky, you reminded us to laugh. You met us when you knew it was too heavy and helped lighten our load. You let us laugh when all we could do was cry.

My Westside community, thank you for loving us, praying, caring, and living faith beside us through this season. You have met the best of life next to the hardest of life and found joy in the midst of it all. You all have been the hands and feet of Jesus. You have carried our entire family and reminded us of grace when we struggled to see it. You were not scared of walking in our brokenness with us. Thank you.

My many, too many, friends who know cancer. You know this story without reading a single word. I love you, and I love that we can speak without sharing a single word. You know. Courtney B Nichols, Jane Coburn, Tim and Suzanne Frye and brave Collin, Alison and Brad Wieker and Luke and LB, Valerie King, Matt and Anna Foral, Mike and Chris Tranier, Luann Snyder, Terra and Kyle Fisk, Becky and Mac McDonald, Donna and Jim Yacovoni, Donna

Kuiper, and the countless others walking with this terrible disease. I pray you are met in each step, walking near to the peace and comfort of Jesus—that in the deep brokenness you would know Jesus anew.

The entire community of administrators and teachers at Evangelical Christian Academy, you have protected and treasured the hearts of our children. Thank you for your ministry to the entire child. We are so grateful. You partnered with us in loving our children big through giant hard. Thank you all.

The staff and families at Latigo Ranch, thank you. You gave us the gift of unforgettable memories together—the best gift this mama could ever ask for—thank you.

Thank you to the endless stream of medical professionals who saw me, loved me, and helped me on this journey. Especially my kind-faced oncologist, Dr. Matthew Logsdon. You have carefully walked me through this journey. Dr. Doug Hammerstrom—you were spot-on when you directed me to him. Thank you. My care has been careful and aggressive when it was called for and quiet when I needed a break. I know it is not easy to see a young mama in such a battle, but you show up, and you care. Thank you for all the medical professionals who see their job higher than a paycheck and more as a calling—your love shows. Thank you.

Shellie Costain, Jen Lints, and Anna George, you fearlessly met the bottom with me. You continue to meet the bottom with me. Brad, Drew, Andrew: thank you for loving your women well as they give so much of themselves in love. And my dear Diana-Autumn Stanley, thank you for loving, for kindness, for living the best of life with babies next to me.

To my daughters in faith, the young ladies who have sat on my pee-soaked purple couch and heard my heart and embraced Jesus and life at its best: Many of the words in this book you have heard me speak. Thank you for coming, for sharing your burdens, for being in my life. Mary Jett, Laura White, Erika Dietrich, Heather McGibbon, Morgan Sellers, Katie Dowdle, Allie Wertenberger, Cosette Kirkpatrick, Ashley Bates. To all the youth who did life next to us, we loved the living with you all. Thank you for giving us entrance into your lives.

Polly and Bill Petro, thank you. Thank you for loving our littles. Thank you for loving us well, supporting us in all seasons of life. Bill, thank you for all your time supporting me with *Mundane Faithfulness.*

Rob Kirkpatrick, thank you for being ready to be present as only you will be able to understand.

Blythe Hunt, you are a treasure, a gift. Thank you for your gift of questions and for helping me develop this part of my book. I love you, and thank you for helping me have a vision of what is to come—the beauty in the brokenness. Aaron Hunt, thank you for being present, faithful, humble, and always reminding Jason and me of grace through your gift of friendship and music. Life is so much better next to you both.

Mickey and Kim Gauen, thank you. Thank you for showing me big love, for inviting me in, giving me a safe place to learn myself. Thank you for your constant love and sacrifice in loving us through chemo and radiation. You extend yourselves in such beautiful love; I'm humbled to know you, to belong to your tribe, and to live better for knowing each of you.

All of you readers who have supported me through this journey and showed up on my blog, *Mundane Faithfulness*, you were often the grace and encouragement that helped me see grace on hard days. Your kindness and endless prayers and support in the telling of my true story have been a gift to my hard days. You have let all the pink have a face. Thank you.

The Megan S. Ott Foundation—you have carried us with your love and amazing generosity. We are humbled to know you in this beautiful awful. You have made this journey a little more bearable for so many.

My people—the people who know all of me. Thank you to my boyfriend and my babies: Jason, Eleanor, Harper Joy, Lake, Story Jane. Life next to each of you is the life I love to live. Thank you for showing grace, extending grace, and walking each day with me. Words fail me when I think of each of you. Each a specific and unique gift I get to love and be loved by in return. You have made my life full, my heart burst with love, and today—this day—amazing.

Finally, Jesus. The Author of me. Thank You for loving this weary, broken woman so well. Thank You for trusting me with the hard in today. Thank You for Your sacrifice for my depraved and broken heart. You died a death I could not, so today, this day, I can walk in grace—proclaiming the greatest story ever told. Your story. Your words made alive in me today. Thank You. Thank You for the life You have given me, and the time to honor and glorify You forever—this life and the next.

How lucky I am to have something that makes saying goodbye so hard.
A. A. Milne, *Winnie-the-Pooh*